HOSPITALISTS' GUIDE TO THE CARE OF OLDER PATIENTS

EDITED BY

BRENT C. WILLIAMS, MD, MPH
Divisions of General Medicine and Geriatrics and Palliative Care
Department of Internal Medicine
University of Michigan

PREETI N. MALANI, MD, MSJ
Division of Infectious Diseases, Department of Internal Medicine
University of Michigan
Geriatric Research Education and Clinical Center
Veterans Affairs Ann Arbor Healthcare System

DAVID H. WESORICK, MD
Division of General Medicine, Hospitalist Program
Department of Internal Medicine
University of Michigan

Series editors
Scott A. Flanders, M.D., SFHM
Sanjay Saint, M.D., M.PH, FHM

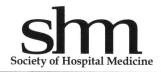

Society of Hospital Medicine

Hospitalists. Transforming Healthcare.
Revolutionizing Patient Care.

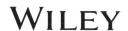

WILEY

Published by John Wiley & Sons, Inc., Hoboken, New Jersey
Published simultaneously in Canada

For general information on our other products and services or for technical support, please
contact our Customer Care Department within the United States at (800) 762-2974, outside
the United States at (317) 572-3993 or fax (317) 572-4002.

Wiley also publishes its books in a variety of electronic formats. Some content that appears
in print may not be available in electronic formats. For more information about Wiley
products, visit our web site at www.wiley.com.

Library of Congress Cataloging-in-Publication Data is available.
978-1-118-12792-6

Printed in the United States of America

10 9 8 7 6 5 4 3 2 1

CONTENTS

CONTRIBUTORS

Esther O. Akinyemi, MD, Department of Psychiatry, University of Michigan; Mental Health Service, Veterans Affairs Ann Arbor Healthcare System

Donna M. Bearden, MD, Division of Gerontology, Geriatrics and Palliative Care, University of Alabama at Birmingham

David C. Belmonte, MD, MS, Department of Psychiatry, University of Michigan

Jolene Bostwick, PharmD, BCPS, BCPP, Department of Clinical, Social, and Administrative Sciences, University of Michigan College of Pharmacy; Adult Psychiatry, University of Michigan

Cynthia J. Brown, MD, MSPH, Division of Gerontology, Geriatrics and Palliative Care, University of Alabama at Birmingham; Birmingham Veterans Affairs Medical Center

Aimée D. Garcia, MD, CWS, FACCWS, Department of Medicine, Geriatrics Section, Baylor College of Medicine; Michael E. DeBakey VA Medical Center

Paul J. Grant, MD, SFHM, FACP, Division of General Medicine, Department of Internal Medicine, University of Michigan

Darius Joshi, MD, CMD, Division of Geriatric and Palliative Medicine, Department of Internal Medicine, University of Michigan Health Center

Christopher S. Kim, MD, MBA, Division of General Medicine, Department of Internal Medicine, University of Michigan Health System

Scott Y.H. Kim, MD, PhD, Department of Psychiatry, Center for Bioethics and Social Sciences in Medicine, University of Michigan

Tia R.M. Kostas, MD, Geriatric Research, Education and Clinical Center, Veterans Affairs Boston Healthcare System; Division of Aging, Brigham and Women's Hospital; Harvard Medical School

Preeti N. Malani, MD, MSJ, Division of Infectious Diseases, Department of Internal Medicine, University of Michigan; Geriatric Research Education and Clinical Center, Veterans Affairs Ann Arbor Healthcare System

Adam D. Marks, MD, MPH, Division of Geriatric and Palliative Medicine, Department of Internal Medicine, University of Michigan

Lauren W. Mazzurco, DO, Division of Geriatric and Palliative Medicine, Department of Internal Medicine, University of Michigan; Veterans Affairs Ann Arbor Healthcare System

Macgregor A. Montaño, PharmD, BCPS, Veterans Affairs Ann Arbor Healthcare System

Joseph Murray, PhD, CCC-SLP, Veterans Affairs Ann Arbor Healthcare System

Satyen Nichani, MD, FHM, Division of General Medicine, Department of Internal Medicine, University of Michigan

Amy B. Rosinski, MD, Department of Psychiatry, University of Michigan

James L. Rudolph, MD, SM, Section of Geriatrics and Palliative Care, Geriatric Research, Education and Clinical Center, VA Boston Healthcare System; Division of Aging, Brigham and Women's Hospital; Harvard Medical School

Lisa S. Seyfried, MD, Department of Psychiatry, University of Michigan

Gabe Solomon, MD, General Medicine, Department of Internal Medicine, Veterans Affairs Ann Arbor Healthcare System

Caroline A. Vitale, MD, Division of Geriatric and Palliative Medicine, Department of Internal Medicine, University of Michigan; Veterans Affairs Ann Arbor Healthcare System

Paul C. Walker, PharmD, FASHP, University of Michigan College of Pharmacy

David H. Wesorick, MD, Division of General Medicine, Hospitalist Program, Department of Internal Medicine, University of Michigan

Brent C. Williams, MD, MPH, Divisions of General Medicine and Geriatrics and Palliative Care, Department of Internal Medicine, University of Michigan

Mark E. Williams, MD, University of Virginia, School of Medicine; Southeastern Area Health Education Center

CHAPTER 1

INTRODUCTION AND OVERVIEW

Brent C. Williams
Preeti N. Malani
David H. Wesorick

Approximately one in three hospitalized adults in the United States is over 65 years of age [1]. With multiple comorbidities and limited physiological and functional reserve, hospitalization inherently represents a period of heightened vulnerability for this population [2]. The risks are clear: falls, delirium, healthcare-associated infections, and adverse effects of drug–drug interactions are common. Even a relatively short period of bed rest can result in profound deconditioning and loss of muscle mass. Between admission and discharge, more than a third of older hospitalized patients experience a decline in activities of daily living (ADLs). Overall, about a quarter of older adults require post-acute care due to loss of independence in basic ADLs and impaired mobility, and a remarkable one-third are rehospitalized within 90 days of discharge [3].

While the risks associated with hospitalization among older patients have been recognized for some time, in recent years significant progress has been made in identifying older patients at highest risk for adverse outcomes, and in structuring interventions to avoid or ameliorate morbidity. Although there is a paucity of research surrounding interventions that improve outcomes in older patients hospitalized on general wards, there is much information from trials among special hospital units (acute care of the elderly, or ACE units), geriatric assessment programs, as well as through intervention programs directed at specific outcomes, such as falls and delirium. A primary purpose of this text is to summarize recent research among hospitalized older patients in a single source, to facilitate incorporation of these findings into hospital practice.

The field of Hospital Medicine has experienced unprecedented growth over the last decade, and hospitalists now provide care for a substantial portion of all hospitalized patients [4]. Although hospitalists treat older

Hospitalists' Guide to the Care of Older Patients, Edited by Brent C. Williams, Preeti N. Malani, and David H. Wesorick.

patients routinely, most have received little or no specific training in the care of older adults. This book attempts to present relevant scientific information about the care of older adults in a way that will be useful to a practicing hospitalist.

INTENDED AUDIENCE AND USE

This book is written for hospitalists—busy clinicians caring for acutely ill patients who need practical, evidence-based information and recommendations to improve the care of the vulnerable elderly. However, we believe other healthcare providers, including nurses, pharmacists, nutrition counselors, and physical and occupational therapists, will find several chapters germane to their work as well.

We also envision this book as a teaching tool, for use especially by hospitalists, medical students, and house officers seeking deeper and more comprehensive assessment and care plans for individual patients, and then embedding new practices into their daily routine.

Each chapter is intended to summarize "best practices"—that is, to provide concise, practical recommendations to hospitalists in the assessment and care of older hospitalized patients based on the most recent scientific evidence. In areas where evidence is scant, authors were encouraged to give practical advice based on their own experience. Topics were selected that addressed areas of high morbidity (e.g., falls, delirium, and medications), controversy (e.g., psychopharmacy and nutrition), or that are particularly difficult to "get right" in a busy hospital practice (e.g., informed decision-making and caring for patients with limited prognosis). Topics for which information and practice recommendations are readily available through other sources, such as management of medical conditions common among older hospitalized patients (e.g., atrial fibrillation, congestive heart failure, and pneumonia) were not included.

We hope hospitalists will use the text in several ways:

- *To build a systematic approach to older patients.* Chapters 2 (Communication and Physical Examination), 3 (Geriatric Assessment for the Hospitalist), 5 (Informed Decision Making), and 13 (Transitional Care Planning) address issues relevant to virtually all older patients, and are applicable in any clinical context.

- *To improve practice in specific contexts.* Many of the chapters address specific clinical contexts (Chapter 9 Hip Fracture, Chapter 10 Falls, and Chapter 11 Pressure Ulcers), and help inform the care of specific types of patients.

- *As a teaching resource.* The chapters in this book are up-to-date, and written by experts in their fields. They are a good starting point for clinical teaching on these topics, and they provide key references that can be used to foster additional reading and discussions.

- *To improve work flow among healthcare team members.* Although our primary audience is hospitalists, in order to be effective, many (if not most) of the recommended practices described in the book require collaborative interactions among physicians, nurses, pharmacists, therapists, social workers, and others. The practice recommendations offered readily lend themselves as a basis to review and redesign local practice with other health team members. Hospitalists who are already involved in quality improvement activities are encouraged to look for specific ideas and practice recommendations to discuss with administrators and other healthcare providers that are most relevant to their own practice environment.

As editors, we learned much from the many talented authors who willingly provided their time and insights to bring this book to fruition. We hope hospitalists and other hospital-based health care providers and administrators will find it equally valuable.

ACKNOWLEDGMENTS

The editors are grateful to our contributing authors, who worked tirelessly to refine text to maximize its usefulness, timeliness, and evidence base, as well as provide expert advice in critical areas where good evidence to improve care is lacking. We are also grateful to Thomas H. Moore, Senior Editor at Wiley-Blackwell Health Sciences, for his thoughtful support and guidance in organizing and compiling the text.

REFERENCES

1. National Hospital Discharge Survey. 2009 table, Number and rate of hospital discharges. 2009. Available at: http://www.cdc.gov/nchs/fastats/older_americans.htm (accessed April 11, 2013).
2. Cigolle CT, Langa KM, Kabeto MU, Tian Z, Blaum CS. Geriatric conditions and disability: the Health and Retirement Study. *Ann Intern Med* 2007;147:156–164.
3. Jencks SF, Williams MV, Coleman EA. Rehospitalizations among patients in the Medicare Fee-for-Service Program. *N Engl J Med* 2009;360:1418–1428.
4. Kuo Y, Sharma G, Freeman JL, Goodwin JS. Growth in the care of older patients by hospitalists in the United States. *N Engl J Med* 2009;360:1102–1112.

CHAPTER 2

THE HOSPITALIZED OLDER ADULT: COMMUNICATION AND PHYSICAL EXAMINATION

Mark E. Williams

INTRODUCTION

Effective interpersonal communication among hospitalists and patients and their families throughout the hospital stay is critical to high-quality care. Good communication can enhance the patient's overall experience, prevent avoidable mishaps and complications, improve diagnostic accuracy and therapeutic efficacy, and foster professional satisfaction. However, the hospital setting is not inherently conducive to effective communication; frequent interruptions, competing demands for physicians' attention, simultaneous tasking, and background distractions of noise and activity are among the myriad barriers. Patients and their caregivers are often anxious and worried about poor outcomes. They feel uncertain about the future and are often groping for some combination of information and assurance that everything will be okay. Despite these challenges, hospitalists can substantially improve communication with patients and their caregivers by applying a few simple principles along with some habits of mind and behavior.

The basic premises of effective clinical care are that clinicians treat individuals not diseases and that the relationship between the doctor and patient is the conduit through which all therapeutic benefits flow. The experienced physician can perceptively gather and integrate clinical information, understand how people behave when they are ill, and develop a plan of care in the patient's best interest. Truly superlative clinical care also requires communicating the necessary therapeutic interventions in a way that maintains and even strengthens the patient–physician relationship. The expert clinician appreciates that he or she is an essential component of the healing

Hospitalists' Guide to the Care of Older Patients, Edited by Brent C. Williams, Preeti N. Malani, and David H. Wesorick.
© 2013 by John Wiley & Sons, Inc. Published 2013 by John Wiley & Sons, Inc.

intervention. Plato stated: "You ought not attempt to cure the eyes without the head, or the head without the body, so neither should you attempt to cure the body without the soul. And this . . . is the reason why the cure of many diseases is unknown to the physicians of Hellas, because they disregard the whole, which ought to be studied also, for the part can never be well unless the whole is well."

PEARLS FOR COMMUNICATING WITH OLDER PATIENTS

Make It a Habit to Demonstrate Reverence for Older Patients

In his classic 1927 *Journal of the American Medical Association* monograph, Francis Ward Peabody said the art of caring for the patient is to care for the patient. He also wrote "The treatment of a disease may be entirely impersonal; the care of a patient must be completely personal." This succinct advice epitomizes the need for craftsmanship in caring.

Caring for patients goes far beyond the important but superficial actions of shaking hands and introducing yourself. For example, we can observe the reverence in how people handle objects they perceive to be extremely valuable. There is a precious delicacy of the touch, with attention to each nuance in movement. The pottery bowl or rare book commands total concentration with an obvious appreciation for the material or artistic value. In the same way, it is easy to identify the clinician who is "caring for the patient" by *how* he or she takes the patient's hand for the initial handshake or to begin the physical examination. Again, there is a sense of conscious appreciation, respect, and reverence.

Control the Environment to Facilitate Communication

Conscientious information gathering requires awareness of the dynamics of the clinical encounter and structuring both the internal and external environment to facilitate communication. This can be particularly challenging in the emergency department or a typical inpatient room. The attitudes and habits of physicians and other healthcare personnel strongly influence the quality of information available from the patient history. In particular, two factors can make all the difference. First, it is important to keep in mind that the overall goals of care are to reduce morbidity and improve function and quality of life by whatever means possible, not necessarily eliminating the cause of the distress (which may be impossible in many circumstances). Second, during the few minutes of each clinical encounter, the hospitalist should develop the habit of clearing clear his/her mind, quieting internal distractors, and paying full attention to the patient through empathic listening. Inattentiveness leads to erosion of the therapeutic relationship and compromises the quality of observations.

Attention to a few specific external environmental considerations can also help by facilitating sensory input to the older person and putting them at ease. Because some older people have visual impairments, techniques to improve nonverbal cues become useful. For example, physicians should avoid having a strong light behind them (such as a window or halogen lamp) because its puts the face in silhouette. Another useful technique is to reduce the distance between participants. As a rule of thumb, the optimal distance is that at which the interviewer begins to feel uncomfortably close. For individuals with hearing impairment, the volume of the voice must be raised without raising the pitch. Shouting, which raises the pitch, defeats the purpose because high-frequency sounds are affected more profoundly than lower-frequency sounds in the aging ear. In fact, shouting can also produce significant discomfort because the failing ear may become more sensitive to loud sounds.

Sit Down and Listen to the Patient

Environmental conditions can improve communication by helping the older patient relax and feel comfortable. One important way to facilitate communication is to sit down. The importance of sitting is inversely proportional to the time available for the encounter; the less the time available, the greater the importance of sitting. Besides providing a common level for eye contact, sitting helps to neutralize the appearance of impatience and haste. The appearance of impatience inhibits communication by magnifying a hierarchical relationship (physician over patient), rather than establishing a partnership to solve problems collaboratively. Sitting down also helps physicians establish the desired internal environment described earlier.

PERFORMING THE GERIATRIC PHYSICAL EXAMINATION

Geriatric assessment begins from the moment the clinician sees the patient and continues until the clinical encounter is complete. The way we wear our hair, the fit of our clothing, what we choose to show off about ourselves and those things we wish to hide are not random. Normally, this self-expression is congruent, and in day-to-day life, we subliminally make a value judgment about the person (pleasant, eccentric, attention seeking, kind, self-centered, etc.) and continue our personal or professional interaction. Incongruities in this self-presentation are important diagnostic clues that require further inquiry. Patients expect to be touched during the physical examination and they are usually acutely aware of the physician's skill, discipline, and thoroughness in gathering clinical data. The importance of this clinical ritual cannot be overstated as an essential part of the therapeutic relationship.

Appearance

The initial appreciation of the patient derives from a broad impression of their body as well as specific features of the individual's uniqueness. These identifying characteristics form the observational basis of our individuality and provide essential clues of the person's inner and outer health. A fundamental question is whether the patient looks acutely ill, chronically ill, or generally well. Does the apparent age (how old the patients looks) match the chronological age? The apparent age may reflect overall health and well-being more accurately than the chronological age. Some nonagenarians look decades younger than their years, and their life expectancy seems to correlate with their apparent age.

The observant clinician notes the patient's body size, shape, and proportions. For example, is the patient overweight or are there signs of weight loss such as temporal wasting or, if more severe, loss of the buccal fat pad? Increases in abdominal fat may suggest the metabolic syndrome with increased risk of diabetes mellitus and premature vascular disease. Skin findings may be obvious over the face, arms, legs, or other areas of exposed skin. Is there the pallor of anemia, the bronze tone of jaundice, the lemon yellow tint of pernicious anemia, the hyperpigmentation of Addison's disease, the ruddy complexion of hypertension or alcoholism, the ecchymosed arm of a recent fall or possible physical abuse? Fresh scars or burns on the upper extremity may be clues to dementia or substance abuse.

No part of the human body is more closely examined than the roughly $25\,in^2$ that comprise the face. Faces are a central focus of our attention, and we are innately attuned to the nuances of those expressions (like joy, fear, pain, anger, sadness, and surprise) that can change with the subtlest movements of the facial muscles. The basic challenge for clinicians is to be able to transcend our usual and preconditioned way of looking at a patient's face to appreciate the individual's nature, as well as their inner state of health. In addition, specific conditions may alter the head and face in characteristic ways (Table 2.1). Pay careful attention to the eyes, the periorbital tissues, and the mouth and surrounding muscles. These parts of the face participate disproportionately in facial expression and communication. Disease predilection also seems to favor these areas.

TABLE 2.1 The Findings of Classic Facies

Condition	Description of facial findings	Other visible clues to the diagnosis
Acromegaly	Prominent jaw; enlarged facial features, especially lips and nose that project away from the head	Large hands with enveloping, pillow-like feel to the handshake
Amyloidosis	Periorbital purpura (raccoon eyes) just after rapid increase in venous pressure from coughing, for example, or, classically, after proctoscopy	Note: raccoon eyes can also be a sign of basilar skull fracture
Cushing's syndrome	Moon face where the buccal fat pads obscure the ears from the front view	Red cheeks
Depression	Worn, weary look; poor eye contact; smile, if present, is forced	Appearance of sadness, loss of pleasure
Klippel–Feil syndrome	Exaggerated forward head position from congenital abnormalities of the cervical vertebrae	
Mitral stenosis	Flushed cheeks; drawn look to the face making nose seem prominent	Exertional dyspnea, atrial fibrillation
Myxedema	Coarse facial features; full, coarse, dry, brittle hair; periorbital edema with little sacs of fluid; loss of the lateral eyebrow; facial puffiness; dull, lethargic expression may be present	Slow movements; large tongue; elbows with dirty-appearing hyperkeratosis
Nephrotic syndrome	Periorbital puffiness; dullness; lassitude	Grayish, sallow pallor if renal failure is present
Paget's disease	Bossing of the forehead causing a large, "Mr. Magoo"-shaped head	Possible hearing aids from deafness
Parkinson's disease	Expressionless, mask-like; slow facial movements, dull eyes peering from upper half of the orbit.	Bent posture; In men, several days of beard growth under the neck because of inability to see this area in the mirror
Polycythemia rubra vera	"Man in the moon face"— concave facial profile resembling a nutcracker doll	

(Continued)

TABLE 2.1 (*Continued*)

Condition	Description of facial findings	Other visible clues to the diagnosis
Scleroderma	Small, tight mouth that may not be fully closed; small oral opening; narrow, pinched nose; shiny skin with minimal wrinkles	Tightening of the fingers, loss of the finger pad
Seborrhea	May be evident in the eyebrows or across the bridge of the nose	Abrupt onset of severe disease suggests HIV infection
Smoking	Excessive facial wrinkles; thin, vertical cracks along the lips; hollow cheeks	Nicotine stains on fingernails
Stroke	Facial asymmetry; facial droop leading to loss of nasolabial fold; droop may include lip	Upper extremity hemiparesis may be present
Tuberculosis	Temporal wasting, malar sweat, loss of the buccal fat pad	Sunken yet bright-appearing eyes

Look carefully at the patient's overall habitus and posture. The hunched forward position of kyphosis reflects previous anterior vertebral compression fractures. The presence of assistive devices such as wheelchairs, canes, or walkers provides obvious clues of impaired ambulation. Musculoskeletal deformities. such as amputations, the arthritic changes of rheumatoid arthritis, the unilateral contractures of cerebrovascular disease, or the frontal bossing of Paget's disease, may be immediately visible.

Notice the presence of adventitious movements. Restlessness can be a worrisome sign in a bedfast or nursing home patient and suggests delirium until proven otherwise. In addition to restlessness, any stereotypic limb movements, such as tremor, chorea, or athetosis provide clues to the person's neurological or behavioral status. Head bobbing from side to side suggests tricuspid insufficiency, while forward and backward bobbing (de Musset's sign) reflects a wide pulse pressure usually from aortic insufficiency. Erratic head movements may suggest an essential tremor. Occasionally, elderly people with severe behavioral problems or psychiatric illness will quietly rock back and forth in their chair.

The presence of makeup in an older woman generally implies well-being or recent clinical improvement if the patient has been ill. Care in the application implies functionally adequate vision and reasonable upper extremity motor coordination. Overapplication may reflect vanity and a strong desire to look much younger. Heavy eyebrow pencil may be an attempt to hide eyebrow hair loss perhaps due to hypothyroidism, systemic lupus erythematosus, syphilis, or heavy metal toxicity. The time of the last hairdo can imply the last time an older woman felt reasonably well. If the patient is wearing nail polish, the distance from the cuticle to the line of polish gives the approximate date of application since nails grow about 0.1 mm/day. Picked-at nail polish can reflect nervousness and agitation.

Dress

Observing the older person's choice of clothing helps in appreciating their state of health, as well as socioeconomic status, personality, culture, and interests. Regretfully, most people seen in the hospital setting are attired in a standard issue hospital gown and not their usual clothing. The interested physician can peruse the reference list for detailed discussions of diagnostic clues from clothing.

Language

The first part of the language assessment is called paralanguage, which deals with the rate and delivery of speech. In essence, paralanguage addresses the manner of speech. How does the patient say what they say? The strength of the person's voice is a useful marker of overall "vitality." This concept can be especially helpful in assessing a familiar patient over the telephone. Illness seems to compromise the patient's voice projection, providing a clue to a change in their status. Paralanguage also addresses the speech rate, pitch, volume, degree of articulation, and quality of the delivery. For example, anxious individuals may speak at a rapid rate at a higher than normal pitch. Soft speech may be a clue to parkinsonism. Another aspect of paralanguage concerns pauses and pause intervals. The pause interval is the time from the end of your utterance to the beginning of the person's response. Normally, this interval varies based on the content. Strong emotionally charged content tends to shorten the pause interval. Unfamiliar content lengthens the interval. If you were asked, "Give me a one sentence summary of the second law of thermodynamics," there might be a pause. If the pauses are always short, we might consider hyperthyroidism, autonomic overactivity, or anxiety. Excessive pause intervals might signify depression, parkinsonism, medication effect, or myxedema.

Another component of language assessment is whether the language makes sense. Can the person communicate a coherent flow of concepts or ideas? Some individuals show digressions from the main theme of the conversation, never returning to the main point. We all know people who communicate this way so a deviation from their normal communication pattern is more revealing than a stable communication pattern. Incomplete thoughts reflect more significant communication difficulty. Does the patient show awareness of the implications of answers (insight), anticipation of an answer, or evidence of abstract thinking? These tend to reflect higher cortical function. Humor does not always indicate higher function unless it is spontaneous to the moment. In fact, some very demented older adults can relate extremely humorous stories from a well-practiced repertoire.

The person's choice of words may be a marker of intellectual vitality. The complexity of syntax also reflects overall education and mental capacity. Specific content issues include evidence or examples of dysfunction; rate of progression; and the nature of adaptations. In evaluating mental status it is useful to see if the person can take a "mental walk" and use their imagination to provide spatial information. For example, "Mrs. Smith, if you met me at the front door of your house and you invited me inside, tell me what we would see." People with dementia have trouble using their imagination and extreme difficulty with this task.

Behaviors

Observing behaviors is easy but interpreting behaviors is a challenge. Nonetheless, some emotions are clearly revealed in gestures. Context is critical in interpreting behaviors. The overall harmony and congruence of the observations are the keys to understanding the meaning of a behavior. Contradictions (apparent incongruities) are very revealing. For example, a nervous laugh can reflect both amusement and extreme discomfort.

The Face

The core of our emotional life is conveyed on the surface of our face. Most details of facial expression are comprised primarily of eye and mouth expressions.

Consider the overall facial expression:

- Is the face animated or flat and masked?
- Are the facial movements symmetric or asymmetric?
- Does the patient seem to be in pain?
- How does the patient use his or her eyes?

Normally, the forehead shows long wrinkles when the person looks up or when the eyebrows raise; absence of this forehead wrinkling suggests thyrotoxicosis or use of Botox. A distinct vertical wrinkle above the eyes in a patient with axial rigidity suggests progressive supranuclear palsy (procerus sign). Cosmetic surgical scars may be visible behind the ear.

The Eyes

Eye movement sends a variety of emotion. For example, eyes that are downcast with the face turned away shows low self-esteem. Gaze aversion can occur if the topic makes one feel uncomfortable or guilty. In grief, the brow is furrowed and the eyes are clenched. The eyes of depression may view the world through partially closed lids. Raised eyebrows suggest disbelief. A sideways glance reflects suspicion, uncertainty, or rejection. Limited eye contact implies the person is hiding something, or perhaps has a low sense of self-esteem. Eye contact can increase if one feels defensive, aggressive, or hostile. Bilateral proptosis suggests hyperthyroidism.

The Mouth

In sadness or depression, the mouth is often stretched and the lip margins may be thinned. The mouth tends to show anger by being tightly compressed. An open mouth with clenched teeth and tightly drawn eyes suggests significant pain. Frowns are easily recognized as signs of displeasure or confusion.

Interpreting smiles is a useful skill to cultivate. The simple smile is open and relaxed, with the mouth pulled up toward the ear and the eyes are slightly closed with a tight lower lid. False smiles tend to be less relaxed with eyes that are open and the corners of the mouth moved lateral rather than up toward the ear.

Arm and Hand Movements

Hand and arm movements are another core element of behavior. Gestures are hand signals that send visual signs of openness, doubt, frustration, inner conflict, and self-esteem. For example, a clenched fist shows determination or aggression.

Sitting and Standing Postures

Sitting on the edge of the bed may imply readiness and a person who is action oriented. Leaning back in a chair with crossed legs while making a kicking movement may reflect boredom and impatience.

A patient's pace, stride, length, and posture can signal emotions and overall vitality. Frail individuals tend to walk slower and without the usual rhythmic cadence. A rapid walk with free hand swing might mean the person is goal oriented. Always walking with one's hands in his/her pockets suggests a person who is secretive, critical, and enjoys playing a devil's advocate role. The elderly person who scuffles with their head down may be signaling dejection. The individual who walks with their hands on their hips denotes sudden bursts of energy. Walking with one's hands behind the back with head bowed and at a slow pace suggests that one is preoccupied. Jingling money in pockets may also reflect preoccupation.

PUTTING IT ALL TOGETHER

The approach to the older adult in the hospital setting requires a different perspective from that needed for the medical evaluation of younger persons. The spectrum of complaints is different; the manifestations of distress are more subtle; the implications for function are more important; and clinical improvements are sometimes less dramatic and slower to appear. The differential diagnosis of common problems is often not the same. Presentations are frequently nonspecific, such as mental status changes, behavioral changes, urinary incontinence, gait disturbance, or weight loss.

Illness versus Disease

Understanding the difference between illness (a person's experience of negative health status) and disease (pathophysiological disorder of one or more organ systems) is a prerequisite to the care of patients affected by incurable disorders. Because older adult patients often present with several chronic diseases, many of which are irreversible, cure-oriented physicians are especially vulnerable to frequent disappointments. The crucial issue is the elderly person's ability to function. Even though many chronic conditions are incurable, the discomfort or disability they produce may be substantially modified. If these concepts are not realized and addressed, elderly patients with irreversible chronic diseases may receive less than optimal care from physicians seeking cures. If we maintain a purely disease-specific focus, we may have difficulty thinking about strategies to best serve the whole patient. Although defining pathological entities may be less complicated than intervening in the illness of the patient, the latter is what constitutes healing.

FURTHER READING

1. Fitzgerald F. The bedside Sherlock Holmes. *West J Med* 1982;137:169–175.
2. Jones TV, Williams ME. Rethinking the approach to evaluating mental functioning of older adults: The value of careful observations. *J Am Geriatr Soc* 1988;36:1128–1134.

3. Peabody FW. The care of the patient. *JAMA* 1927;88:877–882.
4. Verghese A, Brady E, Kapur CC, Horwitz R. The bedside evaluation: Ritual and reason. *Ann Intern Med* 2011;155:550–553.
5. Williams ME, Hadler NM. The illness as the focus of geriatric medicine. *N Engl J Med* 1983;308:1357–1360.
6. Williams ME. Geriatric assessment. *Ann Intern Med* 1986;104:720–721.
7. Williams ME. Sherlock Holmes at the bedside: The case of the missing patient. *J Am Geriatr Soc* 2003;51:1813.
8. Williams ME. *Geriatric Physical Diagnosis: A Guide to Observation and Assessment.* Jefferson, NC: McFarland & Company, Inc., 2008.

CHAPTER 3

GERIATRIC ASSESSMENT FOR THE HOSPITALIST

Brent C. Williams

INTRODUCTION

Two 80-year-old women are admitted to your service one evening to adjacent rooms. Each has had 3 weeks of progressive fatigue and dyspnea on exertion and a chest x-ray showing right middle lobe pneumonia. On admitting examination, each is resting comfortably on 2 L/min O2 per nasal cannula; pulse oximetry shows 96% oxygen saturation. History reveals that they have had well-controlled diabetes and hypertension for 10 years, but no other ongoing medical problems. Physical examination shows findings consistent with pneumonia; you continue oxygen therapy and initiate antibiotic treatment. On the second hospital day, one of the women becomes acutely agitated and confused and falls while attempting to get out of bed, and remains mildly confused throughout her hospital stay, while the second patient has an uneventful admission.

These two patients likely had very different risk profiles for adverse events during their hospital stays, yet had similar medical conditions and presentations. How could the hospitalist have identified the key differences through information gathered at admission? Perhaps more importantly, how can hospitalists approach *all* older patients to: (a) identify the *subset* of patients likely to benefit from additional data gathering (the so-called geriatric review of systems), and (b) gather standardized information for those patients in an efficient manner that is integrated into the standard workflow?

These two questions—how to identify "at-risk" older patients most likely benefit from assessment of domains other than biomedical conditions, such as functional status, caregiver support, and living environment; and how to efficiently gather information most useful in care planning to prevent avoidable morbidity—have been the focus of a broad array of investigations

Hospitalists' Guide to the Care of Older Patients, Edited by Brent C. Williams, Preeti N. Malani, and David H. Wesorick.

over the past 30 years. These assessments are generally termed "geriatric assessment" or "comprehensive geriatric assessment." While few studies have investigated geriatric assessment in the context of usual hospitalists' practices, there is consensus that routinely performing some form of geriatric assessment on selected patients at admission, periodically through the hospital stay, and at discharge is likely to improve patient outcomes.

For the two patients described earlier, the prevalence of clinically significant risk factors is high enough among patients above 75–80 years old to justify some form of geriatric assessment based on their age. Had an assessment been performed, the first patient would have been discovered to have early dementia requiring the assistance of her daughter to manage her meals and finances, and to have fallen twice in the past year, putting her at substantial risk for in-hospital delirium, falls, and infections, and necessitating a brief stay in a skilled nursing facility after discharge. The second patient would have been revealed to participate in 5-km competitive walks on a regular basis, and to be an avid gardener having no difficulties maintaining her daily affairs, placing her at much lower risk for in-hospital or posthospital complications.

The purposes of this chapter are to provide background information on geriatric assessment for hospitalists through a *framework* for geriatric assessment and brief review of evidence regarding comprehensive geriatric assessment, then to provide specific recommendations for applying geriatric assessment in daily practice in hospital medical services.

FRAMEWORK FOR GERIATRIC ASSESSMENT IN THE HOSPITAL

To distinguish risk profiles of the two patients presented at the beginning of the chapter, care of older persons in the hospital setting requires a shift from the traditional acute care model, in which patients are viewed as healthy until struck by an acute illness, to a chronic care model in which an acute illness arises from a background of underlying risk factors and chronic conditions (Fig. 3.1). Unlike the traditional history and physical, which largely focuses on disease- or diagnosis-oriented approaches to assessment, geriatric assessment involves the proactive identification of underlying mental, functional, psychosocial, and environmental conditions and risk factors that affect the health care, quality of life, and outcomes of older patients. As the figure illustrates, an acute illness in an older patient is often the "tip of the iceberg"— an event requiring hospitalization that arises from, or is an acute exacerbation of, underlying conditions. The underlying conditions and context (the "iceberg") that exist before hospitalization, and to which patients return after

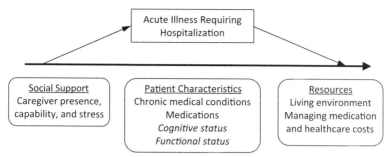

Figure 3.1   Acute-on-chronic framework for hospitalization among older patients.

discharge, are critical determinants of the hospital course and postdischarge outcome for older patients. Aspects of these underlying conditions most relevant to hospital practice fall into three categories—social support, patient characteristics, and resources. Patient characteristics—underlying cognitive and functional impairments (specifically, activities of daily living and gait/mobility) are most immediately relevant to in-hospital and posthospital care. However, managing underlying impairments also requires information on social support (the presence of one or more available and capable caregivers, and the caregiver stress) and available resources (mainly physical living environment and resources to acquire medications and manage healthcare costs). While some background conditions are generally detected by hospitalists (e.g., chronic medical conditions and medications), others are less commonly identified (e.g., caregiver limitations, functional impairment, or a mismatch between functional status and living environment at discharge). It is these background conditions, however, that are often key determinants of patients' risk for adverse events and successful transition from hospital to home.

While detecting and addressing what appears to be a panoply of underlying nonmedical conditions among older patients can appear daunting, keeping this general framework in mind can assist hospitalists in identifying clues to the presence of critical risk factors for adverse hospital or discharge outcomes.

EVIDENCE FOR GERIATRIC ASSESSMENT

With an evidence base developed over 25 years, geriatric assessment has been shown to improve diagnostic accuracy, functional status, placement outcomes, caregiver burden, and survival when applied to appropriately selected individuals.

Comprehensive Geriatric Assessment

Comprehensive Geriatric Assessment (CGA) is "a multidisciplinary evaluation in which the multiple problems of older persons are uncovered, described, and explained, if possible, and . . . a coordinated care plan developed to focus interventions on the person's problems" [1]. The domains usually included in CGA are listed in Table 3.1.

Since the 1980s, dozens of randomized trials of CGA have been conducted in dedicated inpatient units [2–8], at the transition from hospital to home [7, 9–13], and in ambulatory settings [14–19]. Interventions were not standardized, but nearly uniformly included: (a) *selection of frail elders at high risk* for physical or functional decline or hospitalization or nursing home admission, (b) standardized *multidisciplinary assessment and team care planning*, and (c) *longitudinal follow-up* with implementation of a care plan targeted at identified problems. These three principles provide the foundation for the approach to assessing older patients in all settings.

Meta-analyses summarizing the results of randomized trials of CGA [20–23] have shown that CGA decreases nursing home and hospital admissions, improves patients' functional and cognitive status, and decreases overall mortality. However, benefits were observed mainly (though not exclusively) in CGA programs conducted in dedicated inpatient units or around hospital discharge, and in studies completed prior to the early 1990s [20, 22, 24]. In more recent studies and ambulatory settings, benefits have been more difficult to demonstrate, likely due to more widespread incorporation of the principles of comprehensive geriatric assessment in routine practice, and to challenges in selecting only those patients at highest risk for functional decline, nursing home admission, or death.

Acute Care of the Elderly (ACE) Units

Among hospitalized older patients, dedicated geriatric care units that incorporate comprehensive geriatric assessment as routine practice improve patient outcomes. In these units, often termed Acute Care of the Elderly (ACE) units, patient over 70 years of age with acute medical conditions are admitted to a prepared environment to foster patient self-care, multidisciplinary assessment, guideline-based care designed to reduce or avoid functional impairment, interdisciplinary team rounds and discharge planning, and medication review [4, 5]. Patients discharged from geriatric care units have less functional decline, decreased length of stay, and decreased risk of nursing home admission compared with controls. While traditional ACE units are few, given their demonstrated success, many of their features can and should be into the routine care of older patients.

TABLE 3.1 Domains of Geriatric Assessment and Rapid Screening Methods for High-Risk Patients[a] and Target Groups

Domain	Screening questions or assessment
Medical conditions and medications	Routine history and physical exam with medication review
Functional status	
Activities of daily living	Ask: "Do you need help to get going for the day, such as: take a bath or shower, get in and out of bed, go to the bathroom, get dressed, wash face/comb hair/brush teeth?" "Who: (a) does your grocery shopping, (b) fixes your meals, (c) manages your medications?"
Cognition	Perform Mini-Cog [31]: three-item 1-minute recall with Clock Draw or Perform Mini Mental State Examination [32]
Gait/mobility	Ask: "Have you fallen or nearly fallen in the past year?" Perform Timed Up and Go [35]
Urinary continence	Ask: "Do you ever have trouble controlling your urine?"
Self- or caregiver management capacity	
Medication management	Ask: "How do you store your medications at home and remember to take them (pillbox)?" "Tell me a little bit about how you get your (or the patient's) medications."
Social support/caregiver stress	Ask: "Who lives with you?" If dominant caregiver is present, ask caregiver: "What is most challenging about helping to care for (patient)?"
Resources	
Living environment	Ask: "What type of place do you live in?" (house, apartment, assisted living) "Is it difficult getting around in your (house / apartment)?"
Healthcare costs	Ask: "Do you have difficulty paying for your medications?" "What other healthcare costs are most difficult for you to pay for?"
Transportation	Ask: "How do you travel to pick up medications or get to healthcare appointments?"

[a]High-risk patients are defined in Table 3.2.

Geriatric Assessment in "Usual Care" Hospital Services: Hospital Elder Life Programs (HELPs)

In traditional medical and surgical wards, direct evidence for the efficacy of geriatric assessment in the care of older patients is scant. An important exception is the Hospitalized Elder Life Program (HELP), which identifies patients at risk for incident delirium shortly after hospital admission using the Confusion Assessment Method [25]. Protocols to address these risk factors serve to optimize cognitive function (reorientation and therapeutic activities), prevent sleep deprivation, avoid immobility, and treat dehydration. Using these methods, a 40% reduction in incident delirium was achieved [26].

GERIATRIC ASSESSMENT IN HOSPITALIST PRACTICE

Based on the results of the HELP trials and the success of ACE units, the Society of Hospital Medicine [27], the American Geriatrics Society [28], and the British Geriatrics Society [29] recommend routine assessment of high-risk older patients' cognitive and functional status at hospital admission, periodically during the hospital stay, and at discharge [30].

At Admission and During the Hospital Stay

At admission, patients known or suspected to have any of the high-risk criteria listed in Table 3.2 should undergo geriatric assessment. In just a few extra minutes, a wealth of information that informs inpatient orders, and discharge planning can be elicited, following the general outline in Table 3.1.

Functional Status   During the intake history and physical, after completing assessment of the presenting illness, chronic medical conditions, and medications, and before the physical examination, a few additional questions and maneuvers can usually elicit key information, starting with the question "Tell me about your usual morning routine." This engages a conversation about Activities of Daily Living (ADLs) and the need for and presence of caregiver support. Specifically, "Do you need assistance to do any of the following . . ." can lead to a simple listing of the six Basic Activities of Daily Living (getting dressed; brushing teeth, washing face, fixing hair [grooming]; bathing; getting in and out of bed and chairs [transferring]; using the bathroom [toileting]; and eating). Next, key Instrumental Activities of Daily Living (IADLs) can be elicited with three simple questions: "Who does your

TABLE 3.2   Suggested Criteria for High-Risk Patients Appropriate for Geriatric Assessment

American Geriatrics Society [30]
Patients with a history of . . .
   Impairment in basic or instrumental activities of daily living
   Falls
   Urinary or fecal incontinence
   Dementia
   Depression
   Delirium
   Weight loss
   Recent or recurrent hospitalization
   Move to assisted living or nursing home admission under consideration

Authors' additional criteria
Age ≥75
Medical conditions likely to affect functional status (e.g., moderate to severe CHF,
   COPD, peripheral neuropathy; CVA with deficits, visual impairment)

CHF, congestive heart failure; COPD, chronic obstructive pulmonary disease; CVA, cerebrovascular accident.

grocery shopping?", "Who fixes your meals?", and "Who manages your medications?", often with one or two follow-up questions to elicit details.

Cognitive Impairment   Screening for cognitive impairment, if not already clinically obvious, often follows next, and is best accomplished using an assessment instrument rather than history, which is notoriously inaccurate. The transition into formal cognitive assessment is often clumsy or uncomfortable for physicians, but naturally follows IADLs and can be managed with "I'd like to check your memory and thinking next. This is routine for all our patients." Few older patients are surprised or offended by this approach. The examiner can then administer the Mini-Cog [31], which takes about 2 minutes, or the longer Mini Mental State Examination [32]. Steps in administering the Mini-Cog are listed in Table 3.3. It is important to remember that the Mini-Cog is a *screening*, not a diagnostic instrument. A positive test increases the likelihood that a patient is cognitively impaired but is not diagnostic. However, a positive screen may prompt measures to reduce the risk of delirium during the hospital stay and monitor for it presence (described in Chapter 12), and ensure adequate caregiver support and monitoring after discharge.

Gait/Mobility   Although many patients have conditions prohibiting walking at hospital admission, gait should be directly observed whenever

TABLE 3.3   Steps in Administering the Mini-Cog [31]

1. Verify that the patient is able to maintain *attention*. (If not, consider quiet delirium.)
2. Secure adequate lighting and a quiet atmosphere, and ensure that the patient has glasses and hearing aid if needed.
3. Tell the patient you will as ask him/her to say back three words after you have said all three. One- or two-syllable unrelated nouns are used, such as "ball," "pencil," and "airplane."
4. After the patient says back all three words (necessary to indicate the ability to *register* information), state "Now remember those three words, I'll be asking for them again in a minute."
5. Draw a large circle on a piece of paper and tell the patient "I'd like you to draw a clock. Please put numbers inside this circle as you would see them on the face of a clock." Wait without prompting while the patient fills in numbers or completes effort.
6. State "now put hands on the clock to make the time 11:10 (or 8:20)." Wait without prompting until completion of effort.
7. State "Now tell me those three words I asked you to remember." Wait without prompting.

If the patient demonstrates difficulty in accomplishing a task, reassurance may be offered such as "You are doing fine" or "I know this is challenging" but prompts or reminders may not be given.

A *Positive Test* is indicated by *either*: (a) inability to recall any of the three words *or* (b) recall 1–2 words *and* abnormal clock. Clocks may be judged abnormal using common sense inspection.

A *Negative Test* is indicated by *either*: (a) ability to recall 3/3 words *or* (b) recall 1–2 words and a normal clock.

possible. Simply asking the patient to rise from a chair or bed, walk a few steps, and return to the chair/bed to sit down yields a wealth of information on proximal muscle strength, balance, pain during ambulation, and flexibility and joint function. Alternatively, the examiner may ask "Have you fallen or nearly fallen in the past year?", followed by "Are you concerned about falling or take precautions to keep from falling?" Inability or difficulty in performing the maneuver, or a positive response to either question should prompt interventions and monitoring to reduce the risk of in-hospital falls (described in Chapter 10).

Urinary Continence   Identifying chronic urinary incontinence (Table 3.1) can prompt interventions (e.g., timed voids and assistance to the bathroom) to reduce the risk of pressure ulcers and falls from frequent unsupervised trips to the bathroom.

Self-Management Capacity, Caregiver Support, and Resources   A
few brief questions about medication management, transportation, and social
and physical living environment, listed in Table 3.1, will provide key information to ensure that: (a) the people who will be most involved in postdischarge care are included in communication during the hospital stay, and (b)
the patient is discharged to the most appropriate level and type of care
(described in Chapter 13).

As hospital healthcare providers refine and enhance routine workflow
around patient admissions, it is important to remember that many assessment
maneuvers in the intake evaluation, such as functional status assessment,
monitoring for delirium, and falls risk assessment, can be carried out by
nurses or other healthcare providers. However, effective assessment by multiple team members also requires effective, ongoing communication and joint
planning among physicians, nurses, and social workers. Even the role of the
pharmacist in assessing patients to identify and avoid medication-related
complications, of demonstrated effectiveness in ICU settings, is evolving on
general medical and surgical wards.

Discharge Planning (Transition Care)

Many of the same assessment maneuvers performed at admission should be
performed near the time of discharge as well. Directly observing gait is
particularly important at discharge to ensure the use of appropriate assistive
devices, educate the patient and family about mobility precautions and con-
figuring the home for maximal safety, and ensuring the patient is discharged
to the most appropriate care setting (described in Chapter 13).

INTEGRATING ASSESSMENT IN THE HOSPITAL TEAM WORKFLOW

Developing work protocols to identify high-risk older patients, regularly
reevaluate them, and develop targeted discharge plans should involve
continuous refinements to workflow, documentation, and communication
methods among hospitalists, nurses, social workers, and discharge planners.
Hospitalists may work with other healthcare team members and managers
to define routine and special case responsibilities in assessment activities
among physicians, nurses, and social workers. Fully integrating routine
assessment into clinical decision-making will also require developing criteria
for identifying high-risk patients who merit proactive, broader geriatric
assessment; best methods for documentation to make key information available at the time of clinical decision-making; and optimizing communication

among team members on work rounds, electronically, and at team meetings, such as discharge planning rounds. Optimal solutions to these challenges are dependent on local staffing patterns and current workflow among the various healthcare team members, and will vary from hospital to hospital.

Tools to Integrate Assessment into Hospital Care of Older Patients

To facilitate integrating assessment into hospital care, the Society of Hospital Medicine (SHM) has assembled documents describing team care models and assessment and discharge planning processes, and specific screening and assessment tools, termed the Geriatric Care Toolkit (Table 3.4) [33]. Included

TABLE 3.4 Society of Hospital Medicine Geriatric Care Toolbox [33]

Domain	Instruments or resources
General resources	General descriptions of:
	Interdisciplinary teams
	Types of posthospital discharge options
	Functional status assessment
	Drugs to be avoided (specific list)
	Patient/family discharge planning checklist
Mental status	Clock Drawing Test/Mini-Cog
	Confusion Assessment Method (CAM)
	Digit Span Test
	Geriatric Depression Scale(GDS)—Short Form
	Interventions to Prevent Delirium
	Restraint Alternative Menu
	Short Portable Mental Status Questionnaire
Physical function tests	Instrumental Activities of Daily Living (IADLs)
	Physical Self-Maintenance Scale/Activities of Daily Living (ADLs)
	The Functional Activities Questionnaire (FAQ)
Mobility assessment tools	Get Up and Go Test
	Performance Oriented Mobility Assessment
Pain assessment	Pain scales (visual analog or picture)
Pressure ulcers	Braden Scale for Predicting Pressure Sore Risk
	Pressure Ulcer Scale for Healing (PUSH)
Nutrition	DETERMINE (The Nutrition Screening Initiative)
	Nutrition Interventions: Clinical Considerations
	Subjective Global Assessment

are brief instruments to help identify patients with cognitive impairment, delirium and its risk factors, physical function limitations, mobility limitations, pain, and risk factors for pressure ulcers. SHM, with funding from the John A. Hartford Foundation, is now field testing a set of practice guidelines and tools to facilitate transitional care under the Better Outcomes for Older Adults for Safe Transitions (BOOST) program. BOOST provides guidance on analyzing problems in the discharge process and in forming and developing teams to improve discharge planning, assessment tools to identify patients for more intense discharge planning, and templates to provide concise, complete information to primary care providers about the hospital stay [34]. Studies are currently underway to examine the effectiveness of the BOOST program in improving the process and outcomes of hospital discharge for older adults.

CONCLUSION

Through at least the middle of the twenty-first century, hospital care will be transformed by the needs of an aging population. The routine application of geriatric assessment among high-risk older patients to identify hidden morbidities can substantially improve care and care coordination among older adults.

REFERENCES

1. Geriatric assessment methods for clinical decision making. *NIH Consens Statement* 1987;6(13):1–21.
2. Rubenstein LZ, Josephson KR, Wieland D, English PA, Sayre JA, Kane RL. Effectiveness of a geriatric evaluation unit: A randomized clinical trial. *N Engl J Med* 1984;311: 1664–1670.
3. Applegate WB, Miller ST, Graney MJ, et al. A randomized, controlled trial of a geriatric assessment unit in a community rehabilitation hospital. *N Engl J Med* 1990;322:1572.
4. Landefeld CS, Palmer RM, Kresevic DM, et al. A randomized trial of care in a hospital medical unit especially designed to improved the functional outcomes of acutely older patients. *N Engl J Med* 1995;332:1338–1344.
5. Counsell SR, Holder CM, Liebenauer LL, et al. Effects of a multicomponent intervention on functional outcomes and process of care in hospitalized older patients: A randomized controlled trial of Acute Care for Elders (ACE) in a community hospital. *J Am Geriatr Soc* 2000;48:1572–1581.
6. Salvedt I, Mo ES, Fayers P, et al. Reduced mortality in treating acutely sick, frail older patients in a geriatric evaluation and management unit. A prospective, randomized trial. *J Am Geriatr Soc* 2002;50:792–798.
7. Cohen HJ, Feussner JR, Weinberger M, Carnes M, Hamdy RC, Hsieh F, Phibbs C, Lavori P. A controlled trial of inpatient and outpatient geriatric evaluation and management. *N Engl J Med* 2002;346:905–912.

8. Phibbs CS, Holty JE, Goldstein MK, et al. The effect of geriatrics evaluation and management on nursing home use and health care costs: Results from a randomized trial. *Med Care* 2006;44:91–95.

9. Hansen FR, Spedtsberg K, Schroll M. Geriatric follow-up by home visits after discharge from hospital: A randomized controlled trial. *Age Ageing* 1992;21:445–450.

10. Melin AL, Bygren LO. Efficacy of the rehabilitation of elderly primary health care patients after short-stay hospital treatment. *Med Care* 1992;30:1004–1015.

11. Rubin CD, Sizemore MT, Loftis PA, Adams-Huet B, Anderson RJ. The effect of geriatric evaluation and management on Medicare reimbursement in a large public hospital: A randomized clinical trial. *J Am Geriatr Soc* 1992;40:989–995.

12. Naylor MD, Brooten D, Campbell R, et al. Comprehensive discharge planning and home follow-up of hospitalized elders: A randomized clinical trial. *JAMA* 1999;281:613–620.

13. Coleman EA, Parry C, Chalmers S, Min S. The care transitions intervention: Results of a randomized controlled trial. *Arch Intern Med* 2006;166:1822–1828.

14. Tulloch AJ, Moore V. A randomized controlled trial of geriatric screening and surveillance in general practice. *J R Coll Gen Pract* 1979;29:733–742.

15. Williams ME, Williams TF, Zimmer JG, Hall WJ, Podgorski CA. How does the team approach to outpatient geriatric evaluation compare with traditional care: A report of a randomized controlled trial. *J Am Geriatr Soc* 1987;35:1071–1078.

16. Epstein AM, Hall JA, Fretwell M, et al. Consultative geriatrics assessment for ambulatory patients: A randomized trial in a health maintenance organization. *JAMA* 1990;263:538–544.

17. Reuben DB, Frank JC, Hirsch SH, McGuigan KA, Maly RC. A randomized clinical trial of outpatient comprehensive geriatric assessment coupled with an intervention to increase adherence to recommendations. *J Am Geriatr Soc* 1999;47:269–276.

18. Boult C, Boult LB, Morishita L, Dowd B, Kane RL, Urdangarin CF. A randomized clinical trial of outpatient geriatric evaluation and management. *J Am Geriatr Soc* 2001;49(4):351–359.

19. Dorr DA, Wilcox AB, Brunker CP, Burdon RE, Donnelly SM. The effect of technology-supported, multidisease care management on the mortality and hospitalization of seniors. *J Am Geriatr Soc* 2008;56:2195–2202.

20. Stuck AE, Siu AL, Wieland GD, Adams J, Rubenstein LZ. Comprehensive geriatric assessment: A meta-analysis of controlled trials. *Lancet* 1993;342:1032–1036.

21. Kuo H-K, Scandrett KG, Dave J, Mitchell SL. The influence of outpatient comprehensive geriatric assessment on survival: A meta-analysis. *Arch Gerontol Geriatar* 2004;39:245–254.

22. Beswick AD, Rees K, Dieppe P, Ayis S, Gooberman-Hill R, Harwood J, Ebrahim S. Complex interventions to improve physical function and maintain independent living in elderly people: A systematic review and meta-analysis. *Lancet* 2008;371:725–735.

23. Craen KV, Braes T, Wellens N, Denhaerynck K, Flamaing J, Moons P, Boonen S, Gosset C, Petermans J, Milisen K. The effectiveness of inpatient geriatric evaluation and management units: A systematic review and meta-analysis. *J Am Geriatr Soc* 2010;58:83–92.

24. Wieland D. The effectiveness and costs of comprehensive geriatric evaluation and management. *Crit Rev Oncol Hematol* 2003;48:227–237.

25. Inouye SK, van Dyck CH, Alessi CA, Balkan S, Siegal AP, Horwitz RI. Clarifying confusion: The Confusion Assessment Method—A new method for detection of delirium. *Ann Intern Med* 1990;113:941–948.

26. Inouye SK, Bodardus ST, Charpentier PA, et al. A multicomponent intervention to prevent delirium in hospitalized older patients. *N Engl J Med* 1999;340:669–676.

27. Palmer R. Acute hospital care of the elderly: Making a difference. In: *Caring for the Hospitalized Elderly: Current Best Practice and New Horizons. Special Supplement to The Hospitalist.* Philadelphia: Society of Hospital Medicine, 2005, pp. 4–7.
28. American Geriatrics Society. Comprehensive Geriatric Assessment Position Statement. 1998. Last updated August 26, 2005. Available at: http://www.annalsoflongtermcare.com/article/5473 (accessed June 9, 2013).
29. British Geriatrics Society. Comprehensive Assessment for the Older Frail Patient. Best Practice Guide 3.5 (published January 2010).
30. Royer MC, Mion LC Involving the older adult and/or family member in discharge planning. Special supplement to The Hospitalist. 2005. 42–44.
31. Borson S, Scanlan J, Brush M, Vitaliano P, Dokmak A. The mini-cog: A cognitive "vital signs" measure for dementia screening in multi-lingual elderly. *Int J Geriatr Psychiatry* 2000;15:1021–1027.
32. Folstein MF, Folstein SE, McHugh PR. "Mini-mental state": A practical method for grading the cognitive state of patients for the clinician. *J Psychiatr Res* 1975;12: 189–198.
33. Society of Hospital Medicine Geriatric Care Toolbox. Available at: www.hospitalmedicine.org/geriresource/toolbox/project_information.htm (accessed April 10, 2013).
34. Williams MV, Coleman E. BOOSTing the hospital discharge. *J Hosp Med* 2009;4: 209–210.
35. Posiadlo D, Richardson S. The timed "up and go": A test of basic functional mobility for frail elderly persons. *J Am Geriatr Soc* 1991;39:142–148.

CHAPTER 4

INFORMED DECISION-MAKING AND THE EVALUATION OF DECISION-MAKING CAPACITY

Lisa S. Seyfried
Esther O. Akinyemi
Scott Y.H. Kim

INTRODUCTION

Elderly patients admitted to the hospital are at significant risk for having impaired medical decision-making. Ordinarily, adults are presumed to have decision-making capacity (DMC), but this presumption may be challenged when an individual has a condition that impairs the cognitive abilities necessary for making decisions. Hospitalized patients regularly face a wide variety of decisions, such as providing informed consent to a treatment, diagnostic procedure, or discharge plan. Hospitalists must understand how to assess a patient's DMC. While capacity for different decisions must be evaluated independently (rather than a generic "global" capacity), the basic approach is quite similar across contexts (Box 4.1).

The concept of DMC comes from the informed consent doctrine, a principle that is pervasive in modern medicine. Informed consent requires three elements: the adequate *disclosure of information*; *voluntariness*, such that the patient's choice is made free of coercion or undue influence; and *competence*, meaning that the patient has sufficient DMC to use the information given to reach a decision [1]. The terms competence, capacity, and DMC are often used interchangeably, both legally and in clinical practice. If the determination of DMC is made by the courts, it is referred to as "adjudicated."

The need for hospitalists to assess capacity is growing, particularly for those who care for older adults. In 1970, 20% of general hospital inpatients

Hospitalists' Guide to the Care of Older Patients, Edited by Brent C. Williams, Preeti N. Malani, and David H. Wesorick.

BOX *4 . 1*

KEY POINTS

- Decision-making incapacity is common among older patients, and commonly unrecognized by physicians.
- DMC is context specific, not a global patient characteristic.
- Many patients with dementia possess DMC.
  - Cognitive assessment should not be used as a proxy for determining DMC.
- More stringent assessment of DMC is required for patients:
  - Refusing low-risk, high-benefit procedures
  - Requesting high-risk, low-benefit procedures
- Consider court involvement when:
  - Discharge planning for patients unable to care for themselves.
  - Patient disagrees with surrogate. (By law, proxies are usually not permitted to override active objections of patients lacking DMC.)
  - Surrogate decision-maker unavailable, unqualified, or in conflict.
- Beyond strict focus on patients' cognitive capacities for decision-making, clinicians must elicit and incorporate patients' health-related beliefs and values, the role and input of family members, and relevant aspects of specific conditions and symptoms (e.g., nausea and pain) in clinical decision-making.

were aged 65 years and over. By 2006, that percentage had nearly doubled [2]. At the same time, rising healthcare costs compelled hospitals to decrease length of stay, requiring potentially impaired patients to make rapid and often complex decisions. As the population ages and these trends continue, the need for DMC assessment grows even greater. This chapter will address the assessment of medical DMC and some of the nuances associated with the aging population in a practical way.

HOW OFTEN DO PATIENTS LACK DECISION-MAKING CAPACITY?

In the acute care setting, it is not uncommon for patients to lack DMC. The prevalence of patients who lack capacity in the general hospital setting varies from 37% to 48%. The rate of incapacity is higher still in intensive care units

(ICUs) [3, 4]. Despite this high prevalence, clinicians often do not recognize incapacity. Raymont et al. [5] studied 302 consecutive admissions to an acute medical service over an 18-month period. Seventy-two patients (24%) were severely cognitively impaired, unconscious, or unable to express a choice and were automatically deemed to lack capacity. An additional 24% refused to participate or could not speak English. Of the remaining 159 patients interviewed, 31% were judged to lack DMC. They estimated that overall, at least 40% of the patients do not have DMC. They noted that clinical teams rarely identified patients as lacking capacity.

NEUROPSYCHIATRIC CONDITIONS THAT AFFECT CAPACITY

While DMC is often affected in certain medical and psychiatric conditions, a diagnosis does not by itself imply incapacity. However, deficits commonly associated with specific illnesses may impair capacity. Some neuropsychiatric conditions that frequently affect DMC are discussed below.

Delirium

Delirium, an acute dysfunction of cognitive abilities, is a major cause of incapacity in the general hospital setting. For a full description of this important condition, please see Chapter 12. Given that the hallmark of delirium is a fluctuating level of attention and cognition, it follows that a delirious patient may have a diminished ability to utilize sound reasoning and thus have impaired decision-making ability. Despite its high prevalence, few studies have examined the specific relationship between delirium and DMC [4, 6, 7]. In a study of 84 elderly hospitalized patients who developed delirium, Aueswald and colleagues frequently identified a lack of documented informed consent, a lack of cognitive and decisional capacity assessment, and inconsistent surrogate use [7]. In a multisite study of ICUs, more than three-fourths of critically ill patients were unable to provide informed consent throughout their ICU stay with sedation, agitation, and delirium as the most common barriers to consent [4].

Dementia

Dementia, a progressive degenerative disease affecting memory and other cognitive abilities, is common in the elderly, with about 14% of adults over the age of 70 being diagnosed with it in the United States [8]. Cognitive impairment without dementia, termed isolated memory impairment or mild cognitive impairment, is even more prevalent, affecting an additional 22% [9]. The cognitive problems associated with dementia and mild cognitive impairment make patients more likely to have impaired DMC [10, 11]. However, the diagnosis of dementia is not synonymous with incapacity. Depending on the severity of deficits present and the complexity of decision to be made, patients may preserve their ability to make decisions, especially in the early stages of the disease. For example, Kim et al. found that 34% of mild to mild-moderate Alzheimer's disease patients (mean Mini Mental Status Exam 22.9) performed above a threshold validated by a clinician panel on all four standards of DMC [10]. Patients with subcortical neurodegenerative disorders, such as Parkinson's disease, may also develop cognitive impairment leading to diminished decision-making ability [12].

Psychiatric Illness

Psychotic Disorders   Chronic psychotic disorders (such as schizophrenia) are a risk factor for impaired DMC [13]. This incapacity is mainly a function of cognitive impairment and "negative symptoms" characterized by lack of volition, poverty of thought, and concrete thinking. These, rather than the classic "positive symptoms," such as delusions and hallucinations, predispose patients to impaired DMC [14]. This being said, there is wide range of decision-making abilities among people diagnosed with psychotic disorders, and clinicians should not presume these patients to lack capacity. When DMC is impaired in patients with chronic psychosis, understanding (factual comprehension) is usually impaired, while reasoning and appreciation are relatively spared in stable patients. Oftentimes, understanding can be optimized in these patients by a variety of methods to improve DMC. A good rule of thumb is to inquire into the patient's general overall level of functioning—that is, are they permanent residents of a state psychiatric hospital or do they live in the community with some assistance?—as their DMC will tend to correlate with such factors.

Mood Disorders   Mood disorders have varying impact on DMC. Mania, a defining feature of bipolar disorder, is a significant risk factor for incapacity [15]. A manic episode is characterized by impulsivity, distractibility, increased activity, diminished need for sleep, and racing thoughts. It is often associated with poor judgment and psychotic symptoms. While some research has shown repetition can improve understanding in these patients [16], mania remains strongly associated with impaired DMC [17].

Depression may influence DMC, depending on the severity of symptoms. Mild to moderate depression typically has little effect on capacity [18].

Severe depression can have a significant impact on decision-making ability especially when associated with cognitive and/or psychotic symptoms [19].

DETERMINATION OF DECISION-MAKING CAPACITY

All adult patients are presumed to have the capacity to make their own medical decisions. However, this presumption may be called into question when there is sufficient reason for concern. In most states, any physician can assess a patient's capacity to make medical decisions and there is no need for a specialist to conduct the evaluation. Whether a mental health professional should assess a patient's capacity depends primarily on the comfort of the treatment team. Certainly, assessment by a treating physician with the time and knowledge to conduct capacity evaluations has some advantages as he or she has first-hand knowledge of the patient's clinical situation. However, when the evaluation is not straightforward, particularly if an underlying psychiatric condition may be impacting the patient's DMC, consultation with a mental health specialist, such as a psychiatrist or psychologist, may be advisable.

To determine DMC, the following issues need to be addressed (Box 4.2):

1. Is the decision to be made clear?
2. Has adequate information been provided to the patient?
3. Is the patient able to communicate a choice?

BOX 4.2

ESSENTIAL CONDITIONS FOR DECISION-MAKING CAPACITY

- *Physician responsibilities*
  - Nature of the *decision* has been made clear to the patient.
  - Patient has been provided *adequate information* related to the decision.
- *Patient responses*
  - Is able to *communicate* a choice.
  - *Understands* the information provided.
  - Is able to *apply* the information to their own clinical situation.
  - Demonstrates *sound reasoning* abilities.

4. Does the patient understand the information provided?

5. Is the patient able to apply the information to their own clinical situation?

6. Does the patient demonstrate sound reasoning abilities?

The first two questions need to be answered by the treating physician, while the last four questions are to be demonstrated by the patient and are assessed to determine DMC.

Before the Assessment: The Clinician's Responsibilities to the Patient

Valid informed consent requires the adequate disclosure of information to the patient. Thus, it is incumbent on the treating physician to be clear about what decision the patient must make and to provide him or her with sufficient information to make that decision. This may require the physician to obtain more information about the clinical question. For example, a common focus of capacity assessments is determining whether a patient can make a decision regarding disposition from the hospital. If the patient wishes to go home but there is concern that he or she would not be safe, it is not adequate to simply say the situation is "unsafe." It is the responsibility of the treating physician to identify, document, and communicate the specific deficits that will make returning home detrimental.

The patient needs to be provided the following information:

(a) The clinical diagnosis or condition

(b) The proposed treatment or recommendation

(c) The alternatives to the recommended treatment, including no treatment

(d) The risks and benefits of all the options.

The amount and type of information physicians are responsible for disclosing varies by jurisdiction. Some states have a *professional standard* that dictates that physicians disclose the amount of information "a reasonable member of their profession would discuss with patients in a similar situation" [20]. The majority of states use a *patient-centered standard* that dictates the disclosure of what an "average, reasonable patient" would need to know. Once the decision at hand has been clarified and the patient informed, the physician can then assess the patient's DMC.

The modern concept of capacity focuses on patients' function—what they can or cannot actually do [21]. A comprehensive review of court cases, state laws, commission reports, and other ethico-legal literature reveals that the most widely used criteria for capacity, with slight variations, are the following four abilities: communicating a choice, understanding, appreciation, and reasoning [22]. The "four abilities model" has been further defined and informed by empirical data [20] and is the most commonly cited framework for assessing DMC [23].

Communicating a Choice The patient must be able to communicate a clear and consistent choice. Furthermore, the choice must be stable enough to carry out the patient's decision. Communication need not be verbal; if the patient is nonverbal or speaks a different language, steps should be taken to accommodate alternate means of communication such as providing writing materials, using sign language or an interpreter to facilitate communication.

Understanding Understanding is the patient's ability to grasp factual information. This standard is present in all legal definitions of capacity [1]. Understanding entails more than the verbatim repetition of information; the patient must be able to "grasp the fundamental meaning" [24] of the disclosed information. This can be assessed by asking the patient to explain, in his or her own words, the clinical condition, treatment options and associated risks and benefits. Questions such as "Why are you in the hospital?" can help begin the conversation to assess understanding.

Appreciation The ability to appreciate refers to patients' ability apply the disclosed facts to their own situation. Understanding is a prerequisite for appreciation; patients need to first understand their clinical condition and the proposed treatment before they can apply these facts to their individual situation. Questions like "What do you think about your physician's assessment and recommendations?" or "How will this decision affect you?" can help uncover the patient's *beliefs* regarding the facts conveyed to him or her. These beliefs may be substantially erroneous based on prior experience or limited information, or frankly delusional due to an underlying neuropsychiatric or psychotic disorder. For example, a delusional patient may be able to convey a factual understanding of what the doctors said, but then may deny those facts apply to him or her because of a belief that the doctors are actually government agents involved in a plot against the patient.

Reasoning Reasoning refers to the abilities involved in processing provided information leading to a decision. This involves comparing different options, weighing the evidence and drawing logical conclusions. The assessment of a patient's reasoning ability examines the *process* leading to a choice, not how rational the actual decision may or may not be. Essentially, it deals with *how* the patient arrives at the decision and not whether the decision is "reasonable." This can be assessed by asking questions such as, "Tell me what makes you choose this option," and probing the rationale given for their choice.

Applying the "Four Abilities" Model: Considering Function in Context

The modern concept of capacity takes into account both function and context. Determination of DMC must consider both the patient's abilities as well as the circumstances in which he or she must use those abilities. It follows then that cognitive testing should not serve as proxy measure of capacity. Having cognitive impairment does not automatically mean that someone lacks DMC. However, cognitive impairment may alert the physician that a capacity evaluation is warranted. Accordingly, cognitive impairment that sufficiently weakens understanding, appreciation, or reasoning may cause a patient to have diminished capacity.

Capacity Is Task-Specific Just because a patient is able to consent to a medical treatment does not mean that he or she is capable of consenting to a research protocol. A person who is capable of refusing a minor diagnostic procedure may lack the capacity to refuse a life-saving operation. The evaluation of DMC must be task and decision-specific.

Risk–Benefit Ratio Should Be Considered When Setting a Threshold for Capacity It is a widely accepted principle that the threshold for capacity varies according to the risk–benefit profile of the patient's choice [20]. A more lenient standard is applied when a patient is consenting to a low-risk, high-benefit procedure, while a stricter standard is applied if the patient is refusing said procedure. For example, a patient with bacterial meningitis who is agreeing to intravenous antibiotics is held to a different standard of capacity than a hypotensive patient with an active GI bleed who is refusing endoscopy. Similarly, a patient agreeing to a high-risk experimental chemotherapy with little proven benefit is held to a stricter standard than a patient refusing it.

Avoiding a Capacity Evaluation Is Occasionally the Best Course of Action Sometimes, it is possible to avoid the need for a capacity evaluation by changing the context of the patient's decision. Take, for example, a mildly demented man living alone with few supports who refuses the recommendation to go to subacute rehabilitation. Perhaps if sufficient services and resources were put into place, he could return home safely and live independently for a longer time. In this way, the context of his decision is altered in his favor by changing the risk-benefit ratio and making it safer for him to decide to go home.

Documentation of the Evaluation

Documentation of the capacity evaluation has several purposes. First, and most importantly, it justifies and explains the rationale for the capacity judgment. It also serves an educational function, as it summarizes the standards used in capacity evaluation and documents how the determination was made in relationship to the clinical context and abilities of the patient. The documentation of a capacity assessment typically begins with a description of the decision at hand and the reason why a formal evaluation is indicated. A brief summary of the information conveyed to the patient about this choice is helpful, as is a description of the patient's mental status at the time of evaluation. The patient's ability to communicate a choice, understand, appreciate, and reason is documented along with a description of any impairment in these abilities. Lastly, the clinician's categorical judgment about the patient's DMC should be documented, along with the scope of the finding, as a patient may have the ability to make one decision but not another.

CLINICAL IMPLICATIONS OF A CAPACITY EVALUATION DOCUMENT

Assessing capacity may be challenging in some cases, but even more challenging sometimes are the clinical implications of the outcome of the assessment. When a patient is deemed to have capacity, the patient is then allowed to make his or her own decisions, even to their own detriment. This may be frustrating to the medical team who is charged with providing emergency care even when patient has refused to comply with previous recommendations. For example, a patient who chronically abuses alcohol with a history of delirium tremens may present frequently to the emergency room for alcohol withdrawal treatment but refuse to engage in more definitive substance use treatment once he is sober. Even when the patient is deemed to lack the capacity, the clinical decision will often require at least the assent of the patient for success to occur. For example, a delirious patient who needs a feeding tube but adamantly refuses it may sabotage the treatment even when the decision to proceed is made by a surrogate decision-maker. It then becomes important to determine what utility a capacity assessment will serve the patient and whether it may be of more benefit to address the patient's concerns and work within his or her expectations.

Who Is the Surrogate Decision-Maker?   When a patient is deemed incapacitated, it becomes important to consider the issue of a surrogate decision-maker. It is important however to consider the following questions: (a) Is the lack of capacity temporary or permanent? (b) Is the decision to be made emergent, urgent, or routine? If a patient lacks capacity temporarily and a routine decision needs to be made, the patient's capacity should be optimized and the decision deferred until the patient regains capacity. Patients lacking capacity, either permanently or temporarily, who need to make a decision urgently require a surrogate decision-maker, such as a durable power of attorney (DPOA), next of kin, or a temporary legal guardian. The appropriate ranking of next-of-kin differs from jurisdiction to jurisdiction. The order in most laws is typically spouse, adult child, parent, sibling, then usually nearest relative but sometimes a close friend. Some states also mention life partners as taking the place of "spouse" in the hierarchy. Practically speaking, clinicians often find themselves interacting with the next of kin who are the most available and invested but who may not be the designated decision-maker indicated by the hierarchy. This is appropriate as long as the team has done the due diligence to find and involve the designated next kin. If there is no available surrogate decision-maker, and time does not allow for a temporary guardian to be appointed, then the decision may be made by physicians as to what is in the "best interest" of the patient. In the hospital setting, this is usually done in conjunction with an ethics committee. For patients whose incapacity will likely be chronic, a more permanent surrogate is recommended. Guardianship should be sought when other mechanisms for surrogate decision-making are not available for an incapacitated patient who is likely to face a series of major medical decisions.

When to Involve the Courts   While the vast majority of DMC evaluations are incorporated into the routine medical decision-making for the patient, there are some cases that require review by the courts.

Inability to Care for Oneself   One of the most common reasons for going to court is when an elderly patient who has been living alone can no longer do so safely but is refusing placement in a living facility. A patient with significant dementia may have previously functioned at home with the help of his wife but, after she dies, he may no longer be safe at home. If he insists on returning home to an unsafe setting and is found to lack the capacity to decide on his disposition, the hospital may have no choice but to go to court. Ideally, a caring family member would petition for guardianship, but if the patient has no family members, the hospital may need to petition the court to appoint a guardian.

Patient Disagrees with Surrogate or the Clinical Determination of Incompetence   Most healthcare proxy laws do not authorize a proxy to override the active objection of a patient even if the patient has been deemed to lack capacity by a physician. In addition, if a patient disagrees with the clinical determination of incompetence, the issue may need to be settled by the courts.

Surrogate Decision-Maker Is Not Available, Is Unqualified, or Is in Conflict   When the surrogate decision-maker is not able to carry out his or her duties—whether this person is a de facto surrogate, a health care proxy, a durable power of attorney for health care, or even a guardian, the courts may need to appoint an alternative decision-maker. For example, the surrogate may himself be impaired or may have a conflict of interest. When there are intractable conflicts among potential surrogates, courts may have to decide who will have the final decision-making authority for the patient. For patients without a formally designated surrogate, such as a healthcare proxy, most states have some type of de facto surrogate treatment laws that guide practice.

BEYOND CAPACITY ASSESSMENT: WORKING WITH PATIENTS MAKING DECISIONS

Decision-making must be considered from a clinical standpoint, not simply a legal one. The clinician's job is not finished once the determination of capacity is made. Even when a patient is found to be competent to make his or her own decisions, there are important aspects of decision-making of which the clinician should be aware.

Influences on Medical Decision-Making

The cognitive aspects involved in decision-making are typically of most concern to clinicians. Yet the decision-making process can be influenced by factors that are not rational but, rather, processes that are unconscious or driven by emotion. These broader influences should be considered as part of a patient's overall clinical picture as they are part of the context in which patients make their choices.

Race, Ethnicity, and Culture   As the elderly population grows, so does its racial and ethnic diversity. Between 2010 and 2030, the number of older minorities is projected to increase by 160% as compared with 59% in the white population [25]. As such, it becomes increasingly important to understand the impact that race or ethnicity and culture can have on medical decision-making. For example, a growing body of research suggests that these factors have significant effects on end-of-life decision-making. African-Americans and Hispanic-Americans are more likely to prefer the use of life support as compared with white patients [26]. Many non-Western cultures prefer not to burden the patient with decisions and emphasize a family-centered model of medical decision-making [27].

Personal Values   While it may seem obvious that personal values play a significant role in decision-making, clinicians may not always elicit an individual's values. Values are often not systematically assessed during capacity evaluations, although some of the issues relating to values may be uncovered when appreciation and reasoning are being evaluated [20, 28]. Karel et al. have identified three dimensions of personal healthcare values that may be useful to elicit when guiding a patient through the decision-making process: (a) personal perspectives on quality of life in terms of one's abilities, activities, and relationships; (b) beliefs on preserving quality versus length of life; and (c) preferences for one's role in decision-making [29]. Older patients often prefer to have family members or physicians involved in the decision-making process [30].

Family Considerations   Patients' decisions are often influenced by their personal relationships. As such, an understanding of the patient's family dynamic can be quite useful. The amount of family involvement varies from patient to patient. Some families are very involved in medical decision-making—taking an active role in discussions about treatment and helping the patient reach a decision. Other families are involved only indirectly, but their involvement might be important to the patient [31]. The treating clinician should elicit the patient's preferences in this regard and offer to have the patient's family present during discussions if he or she so desires. Families can have strong opinions and may pressure the patient to make a particular decision. While this could be interpreted as a threat to "voluntariness," it is more useful to think of these pressures as part of the context in which the patient is making decisions [20].

Obstacles to Good Decision-Making

Consider a situation in which a competent patient refuses a high-potential-benefit, low-risk intervention. The law is clear on what the clinician must do; respect the patient's autonomy and honor his choice to decline treatment. Yet a clinician must be careful not to abandon the patient to his or her rights.

There is a professional obligation beyond simply doing whatever the patient wants. The clinician is charged with respecting and promoting patient self-determination and this means ensuring what the patient decides is *truly* what he or she wants. A patient in severe pain that is undertreated may refuse an intervention. But is that refusal truly an autonomous, considered decision? Pain is just one of many obstacles to good decision-making that patients may encounter in the hospital. There are many other burdensome symptoms, such as nausea, shortness of breath, insomnia, and constipation that the clinician must adequately manage. Patients may also have psychiatric conditions that are unrecognized or undertreated. A patient's symptoms of severe depression may go unaddressed as many (fatigue, apathy, poor sleep, and appetite) are also common to serious medical illnesses. Patients with personality disorders often have difficulty coping with their medical situation and may behave in self-destructive and/or antagonizing ways that anger and confuse their treatment teams. A psychiatric consult may help manage these situations.

CONCLUSION

The evaluation of treatment consent must be considered from a clinical, not just legal, perspective. Treating clinicians should take an active role in identifying and removing barriers to decisional capacity. That role may include resolving the problem that prompted the question of incapacity in the first place (a patient may refuse a recommended treatment because of ongoing pain or other burdensome symptoms). It may involve enhancing a patient's consent capacity though further education. Ultimately, that role may involve fostering a competent patient's autonomy when faced with a difficult decision.

REFERENCES

1. Berg JS, Appelbaum PS, Parker LS, Lidz CW. *Informed Consent: Legal Theory and Clinical Practice*. New York: Oxford University Press, 2001.
2. DeFrances CJ. 2006 National Hospital Discharge Survey. National Health Statistics Reports. 2008(5):1–20.
3. Cohen LM, McCue JD, Green GM. Do clinical and formal assessments of the capacity of patients in the intensive care unit to make decisions agree? *Arch Intern Med* 1993;153(8):2481–2485.
4. Fan E, Shahid S, Kondreddi VP, Bienvenu OJ, Mendez-Tellez PA, Pronovost PJ, et al. Informed consent in the critically ill: A two-step approach incorporating delirium screening. *Crit Care Med* 2008;36(1):94–99.
5. Raymont V, Bingley W, Buchanan A, David AS, Hayward P, Wessely S, et al. Prevalence of mental incapacity in medical inpatients and associated risk factors: Cross-sectional study. *Lancet* 2004;364:1421–1427.

6. Adamis D, Martin FC, Treloar A, Macdonald AJ. Capacity, consent, and selection bias in a study of delirium. *J Med Ethics* 2005;31(3):137–143.

7. Auerswald KB, Charpentier PA, Inouye SK. The informed consent process in older patients who developed delirium: A clinical epidemiologic study. *Am J Med* 1997; 103(5):410–418.

8. Plassman BL, Langa KM, Fisher GG, Heeringa SG, Weir DR, Ofstedal MB, et al. Prevalence of dementia in the United States: The aging, demographics, and memory study. *Neuroepidemiology* 2007;29(1–2):125–132.

9. Plassman BL, Langa KM, Fisher GG, Heeringa SG, Weir DR, Ofstedal MB, et al. Prevalence of cognitive impairment without dementia in the United States. *Ann Intern Med* 2008;148(6):427–434.

10. Kim SYH, Caine ED, Currier GW, Leibovici A, Ryan JM. Assessing the competence of persons with Alzheimer's disease in providing informed consent for participation in research. *Am J Psychiatry* 2001;158:712–717.

11. Okonkwo O, Griffith HR, Belue K, Lanza S, Zamrini EY, Harrell LE, et al. Medical decision-making capacity in patients with mild cognitive impairment. *Neurology* 2007; 69(15):1528–1535.

12. Dymek MP, Atchison P, Harrell L, Marson DC. Competency to consent to medical treatment in cognitively impaired patients with Parkinson's disease. *Neurology* 2001;56(1): 17–24.

13. Grisso T, Appelbaum PS, Mulvey EP, Fletcher K. The MacArthur Treatment Competence Study. II: Measures of abilities related to competence to consent to treatment. *Law Hum Behav* 1995;19(2):127–148.

14. Palmer BW, Dunn LB, Depp CA, Eyler LT, Jeste DV. Decisional capacity to consent to research among patients with bipolar disorder: Comparison with schizophrenia patients and healthy subjects. *J Clin Psychiatry* 2007;68(5):689–696.

15. Owen GS, Richardson G, David AS, Szmukler G, Hayward P, Hotopf M. Mental capacity to make decisions on treatment in people admitted to psychiatric hospitals: Cross sectional study. *BMJ* 2008;337:a448.

16. Misra S, Socherman R, Park BS, Hauser P, Ganzini L. Influence of mood state on capacity to consent to research in patients with bipolar disorder. *Bipolar Disord* 2008;10(2): 303–309.

17. Beckett J, Chaplin R. Capacity to consent to treatment in patients with acute mania. *Psychiatr Bull* 2006;30(11):419–422.

18. Vollmann J, Bauer A, Danker-Hopfe H, Helmchen H. Competence of mentally ill patients: A comparative empirical study. *Psychol Med* 2003;33:1463–1471.

19. Lapid MK, Rummans TA, Poole KL, Pankratz S, Maurer MS, Rasmussen KG, et al. Decisional capacity of severely depressed patients requiring electroconvulsive therapy. *JECT* 2003;19(2):67–72.

20. Grisso T, Appelbaum PS. Assessing Competence to Consent to Treatment: A Guide for Physicians and Other Health Professionals. London: Oxford University Press, 1998.

21. Grisso, T. *Evaluating Competencies: Forensic Assessments and Instruments*, 2nd ed. New York: Kluwer/Plenum, 2003, pp. 23–28.

22. Berg JW, Appelbaum PS, Grisso T. Constructing competence: Formulating standards of legal competence to make medical decisions. *Rutgers Law Rev* 1996;48:345–396.

23. Kim SYH. Evaluation of Capacity to Consent to Treatment and Research. New York: Oxford University Press, 2010.

24. Appelbaum PS. Assessment of Patients' Competence to Consent to Treatment. *NEJM* 2007;357:1834–1840.

25. Administration on Aging, Department of Health and Human Services. Profile of Older Americans: 2010. Available at: http://www.aoa.gov/aoaroot/aging_statistics/Profile/2010/4.aspx (accessed April 11, 2013).

26. Kwak J. Current research findings on end-of-life decision making among racially or ethnically diverse groups. *Gerontologist* 2005;45(5):634–641.

27. Blackhall LJ. Ethnicity and attitudes toward patient autonomy. *JAMA* 1995;274(10): 820–825.

28. Appelbaum PS. Ought We to require emotional capacity as part of decisional competence? *Kennedy Inst Ethics J* 1998;8(4):377–387.

29. Karel MJ. Reasoning in the capacity to make medical decisions: The consideration of values. *J Clin Ethics* 2010;21(1):58–71.

30. Hornung CA. Ethnicity and decision-makers in a group of frail older people. *J Am Geriatr Soc* 1998;46(3):280–286.

31. Gilbar R. Family involvement, independence, and patient autonomy in practice. *Med Law Rev* 2011;19(2):192–234.

CHAPTER 5

CARING FOR PATIENTS WITH LIMITED PROGNOSIS: NEGOTIATING GOALS OF CARE AND PLANNING FOR THE END-OF-LIFE

Adam D. Marks
Caroline A. Vitale

INTRODUCTION

Despite data showing that goals of care discussions are associated with both improved patient satisfaction and increased concordance between patient's wishes and the care received, physicians often shy away from discussions about end of life issues. The nature of hospital medicine in general, characterized by short hospital stays that tend to be focused on acute events rather than "big-picture" models of care, does not foster the type of doctor–patient relationships that encourage such talks. However, given that a significant proportion of older adults are hospitalized (often multiple times) in the years or months prior to death, hospitalists may actually find themselves in an optimal position to talk to hospitalized patients and their families about their goals and wishes, allowing for realistic, "in-the-moment" decision-making [1].

Although the ability to discuss prognosis and negotiate goals of care are essential skills needed in caring for hospitalized patients of any age, these skills are especially important for those providers caring for the growing number of frail older adults hospitalized each year. As more people live to later years, the number of older adults accumulating multiple chronic illnesses has increased, leading to a protracted course of progressive disability and eventual death. This progression towards the end of life is often

Hospitalists' Guide to the Care of Older Patients, Edited by Brent C. Williams, Preeti N. Malani, and David H. Wesorick.

characterized by multiple hospitalizations, invasive procedures, and significant morbidity. Although the majority of older adults wish to de-escalate care
at the end of life, in 2006 more than 25% of Medicare spending went to
patients in the last year of their life; of that 25%, almost 80% of costs were
incurred in the final month of life [2].

In this chapter, we will review the unique challenges facing geriatric
patients with limited prognosis; the core concepts of palliative and hospice
care; existing concepts and tools of prognostication in the elderly; techniques
to facilitate goals of care discussion; and the means by which effective planning for end-of-life care can occur. Our goal is to provide the hospitalist with
practical guidance surrounding these important aspects of comprehensive
care for the older patient.

ROLE OF PALLIATIVE CARE IN THE CARE OF PATIENTS WITH LIMITED PROGNOSIS

Broadly speaking, palliative care refers to any care that is not curative in
intent. While several formal definitions exist, the 2002 World Health Organization (WHO) definition has been widely adopted and describes palliative
care as:

> an approach that improves the quality of life of patients and their fami-
> lies facing the problems associated with life-threatening illness, through
> the prevention and relief of suffering by means of early identification
> and impeccable assessment and treatment of pain and other problems,
> physical, psychosocial and spiritual.

Palliative care does not need to be limited to patients at the end of life.
In fact, emerging research indicates that improved outcomes are associated
when palliative care is pursued earlier in the disease course [3].

The basic tenets of palliative care include an emphasis on symptom
relief, respect for patient's goals of care, and the maintenance of dignity
during the course of a patient's disease process. Such an approach does not
exclude curative therapies; indeed, an ideal palliative approach would be
applied to all patients with complex and life-limiting disease (Fig. 5.1).

A great deal of confusion exists among patients and healthcare professionals about the difference between palliative care and hospice. Palliative
care, as defined above, can be appropriately applied to many patients with
life-limiting conditions long before they approach the end of life. Hospice,
on the other hand, traditionally refers to the services provided for patients
who are estimated to have a life expectancy of less than 6 months. Hospice
will be discussed more fully towards the end of this chapter.

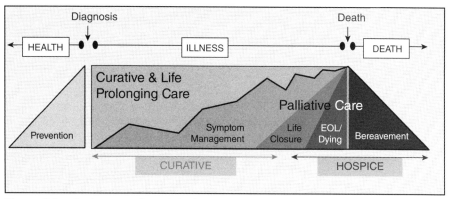

Figure 5.1   An integrated model of palliative care. This model of care emphasizes the coadministration of curative and palliative care across the spectrum of disease. Adapted from the World Health Organization Report on Cancer Pain and Palliative Care, reproduced with permission [4]. (See color insert.)

ASSESSING PROGNOSIS

> As a result of a failure to prognosticate, let alone prognosticate accurately, patients may die deaths they deplore in locations they despise.
> —Christakis [5]

Effective prognostication has been shown to be a key factor for patient and families as they discuss goals of care and end of life planning, and is a common question for healthcare providers when breaking news of a terminal diagnosis. Indeed, it is difficult to discuss goals of care and formulate a plan for end of life care without a shared understanding of a patient's general prognosis. Clinicians, however, have traditionally demonstrated a limited ability to accurately prognosticate, often overestimating survival by two- to fivefold [5]. Furthermore, the inherent likelihood for older adults to have multiple comorbidities that affect outcome (e.g., chronic renal insufficiency, dementia, and debility) can further frustrate efforts to provide accurate information for patients and families. Interestingly, research suggests that a closer doctor–patient relationship is associated with more optimistic and less accurate prognostication; thus, the argument could be made that hospitalists, with their more limited relationship to patients, might be better prognosticators than other health care professionals.

Although arbitrary, identifying those patients with an estimated prognosis of less than 6 months is of practical importance since these patients would qualify for hospice services. Thus, the majority of research on models of prognosis has involved estimating which patients have less than 6 months

TABLE 5.1   Online Resources for Prognostication

General Prognosis in Older Adults:
  http://www.eprognosis.org
Estimating Prognosis in Advanced Dementia (Mortality Risk Index—MRI):
  http://www.eperc.mcw.edu/EPERC/FastFactsIndex/ff_150.htm
Congestive Heart Disease Prognosis Tool:
  http://depts.washington.edu/shfm/app.php
Risk of a Cardiovascular Event:
  http://depts.washington.edu/shfm/app.php
Cancer Prognosis Tools:
  http://www.mskcc.org/cancer-care/prediction-tools
  https://www.adjuvantonline.com/index.jsp
  http://www.predict.nhs.uk/
  http://www.personalizedrx.org:8080/OnlineTool/
Chronic Obstructive Pulmonary Disease Prognosis Tool:
  http://www.qxmd.com/calculate-online/respirology/bode-index

to live and have focused primarily on patients with advanced cancer. Fittingly, metastatic cancer has the most easily predictable course among common life-limiting illnesses. In comparison, other progressive conditions, such as congestive heart failure (CHF) or chronic obstructive pulmonary disease (COPD), often have courses characterized by acute exacerbations followed by a period of stabilization. Predicting survival in these cases is often much more problematic, as it can be unclear during an acute exacerbation whether the patient will return to their baseline functioning or will instead progress to active dying. Using techniques similar to those used in neoplastic processes, prognostic models have been developed for a variety of conditions, including CHF, COPD, and liver failure (Table 5.1). While it is beyond the scope of this chapter to review the utility of each model, we will briefly mention those used most commonly, and focus on models of prognosis for dementia and debility, as both are common conditions under which patients can often meet hospice admission criteria.

GENERAL CONCEPTS OF PROGNOSIS

The cornerstone of accurate prognosis is accurate diagnosis and evaluation of the extent of disease. Thus, even in cases where treatment options are limited for other reasons (debility, comorbid conditions) diagnostic measures may be appropriate to provide the patient and family with useful prognostic information. That said, the potential benefit of a diagnosis must be weighed against the risk of the diagnostic procedure(s) being considered.

Patients' prognosis depends not only on their primary diagnosis, but on a host of other factors, including functional status, nutritional status, and number and severity of comorbid conditions. Functional status, in particular, has been shown to strongly affect prognosis in a variety of conditions, from cancer to dementia. Several tools for assessing functional status have been used to aid in prognostication, the most widely used of which include the Eastern Cooperative Oncology Group (ECOG) Performance Score and the Karnofsky score, which are derived from cancer populations. A more useful scale that has been studied in both cancer and noncancer populations, as well as in older adults, is the Palliative Performance Scale (Table 5.2). This scale may be more applicable to older adults as it incorporates ambulatory status along with level of alertness and nutritional intake.

Regarding nutritional status, several markers are traditionally used to aid in prognostication and are often informally taken into account when determining whether a patient meets hospice criteria, though evidence behind these measures are often lacking (see Chapter 8). These include serum albumin, changes in weight, and presence or absence of aspiration pneumonia. A serum albumin less than 2.5 mg/dL, weight loss greater than 10% during the past 6 months, and recurrent aspiration pneumonia are considered risk factors for a prognosis of less than 6 months among patients with dementia and debility (see below) and can help determine hospice eligibility.

TOOLS USED IN PROGNOSIS: DEBILITY AND DEMENTIA

Debility

During the past few years, increasing attention has been paid to the concept of debility (also known as progressive frailty or geriatric failure to thrive) in relation to prognosis among geriatric populations. This concept refers to the growing subset of patients who do not die of one specific terminal condition; rather, these patients experience a progressive decline that is characterized by multiple comorbidities and progressively impaired physical function and/or cognition. The decline is by definition not related to a single identifiable cause, and such a diagnosis should only be made after reversible causes are ruled out. Despite the lack of any validated, universally accepted criteria, the National Hospice and Palliative Care Organization (NHPCO) has developed general criteria for hospice admission under which those older adults with non-cancer diagnoses who do not fall into one of the condition-specific

TABLE 5.2 Palliative Performance Scale [6]

%	Ambulation	Activity level / Evidence of disease	Self-care	Intake	Level of consciousness	Estimated median survival in days		
						(a)	(b)	(c)
100	Full	Normal / *No disease*	Full	Normal	Full	N/A	N/A	108
90	Full	Normal / *Some disease*	Full	Normal	Full			
80	Full	Normal with effort / *Some disease*	Full	Normal or reduced	Full			
70	Reduced	Cannot do normal job or work / *Some disease*	Full	As above	Full	145		
60	Reduced	Cannot do hobbies or housework / *Significant disease*	Occasional assistance needed	As above	Full or confusion	29	4	
50	Mainly sit/lie	Cannot do any work / *Extensive disease*	Considerable assistance needed	As above	Full or confusion	30	11	41
40	Mainly in bed	As above	Mainly assistance	As above	Full or drowsy or confusion	18	8	
30	Bed bound	As above	Total care	Reduced	As above	8	5	
20	Bed bound	As above	As above	Minimal	As above	4	2	6
10	Bed bound	As above	As above	Mouth care only	Drowsy or coma	1	1	
0	Death	–	–	–	–			

Survival postadmission to an inpatient palliative unit, all diagnoses
Days until inpatient death following admission to an acute hospice unit, diagnoses not specified
Survival postadmission to an inpatient palliative unit, cancer patients only

TABLE 5.3   Hospice Enrollment Criteria for Debility [7]

Patients over the age of 65 may qualify for hospice services, independent of other terminal diagnoses, if they have the following:
- Decreasing weight >10% over the past 6 months
- Albumin <2.5, with a decrease over the past 6 months
- Loss of functional status, including increasing dependence of ADLs
- Dysphagia leading to recurrent aspiration or chronic inadequate nutritional intake
- Progressive pressure ulcers despite appropriate nursing and wound care
- Increasing need for emergency visits or hospitalizations related to the chronic medical conditions (CHF, COPD, etc.)

criteria may still qualify for hospice enrollment. Patients in this category meet the "debility criteria" for enrollment that take several factors into account (Table 5.3). While efforts are ongoing to validate these criteria across different geriatric populations, they can serve as a general guide to practitioners in their efforts to provide accurate prognostic information. It is important to note that while frail, older adults may not meet strict criteria for hospice, many of these individuals often benefit from a palliative approach to their care, with an emphasis on quality of life rather than aggressive life-prolonging measures.

Dementia

As with debility, the diagnosis of dementia is increasingly recognized as a progressive, life-limiting disease. The difficulty in identifying dementia as a terminal condition is a major barrier to the utilization of palliative care and hospice services for this patient population. In recent years, extensive work has been done to develop tools that can accurately predict 6-month mortality among dementia patients. To date, there are no "gold standard" criteria by which a patient with dementia can be determined to have a prognosis of less than 6 months. However, the NHPCO has based the dementia hospice eligibility criteria on the Functional Assessment Staging (FAST) [8]. According to the NHPCO guidelines, a stage of at least 7A (loss of ambulation, loss of vocabulary to <6 words) is appropriate for hospice enrollment (Table 5.4). Data regarding the predictive prognostic value of the FAST system, however, is limited.

More recently, the Mortality Risk Index (MRI) (Table 5.1) has been suggested as an alternative to FAST [9]. Developed in 2004, the MRI was evaluated among newly admitted nursing home residents and has been used

TABLE 5.4   Hospice Enrollment Criteria for Dementia [7]

Patients with a diagnosis of dementia may qualify for hospice services, independent of other terminal diagnoses, if the following criteria are met:
- FAST Stage 7A or greater (ability to speak limited to six words)
- Impaired function, characterized by:
  - Inability to ambulate
  - Inability to bathe/dress without assistance
  - Incontinent of urine and/or stool.
- One of the following six medical complications:
  - Aspiration pneumonia
  - Upper urinary tract infection
  - Progressive decubitus ulcers despite appropriate wound care
  - 10% weight loss in the past 6 months not related to reversible cause
  - Septicemia
  - Fever recurrent with antibiotics.

by some to predict mortality in patients with advanced dementia utilizing clinical parameters, such as the presence of shortness of breath, amount of time awake, amount of food eaten at meals, in addition to functional status. In this population, the MRI was found to have a greater predictive value of 6-month prognosis when compared with the FAST. However, additional research is needed regarding the validity of applying these measures to the broader geriatric population.

COMMUNICATION WITH PATIENT AND FAMILIES REGARDING PROGNOSIS AND NEGOTIATING GOALS OF CARE

Effective communication with patient and families is a key component of medical care across disciplines, and is associated with improved patient satisfaction and decreased patient anxiety and distress (see Chapter 3). Compared with other domains, the inherent fear and uncertainty associated with discussions of life-threatening or life-limiting illness adds an emotional element that can make effective communication more difficult. In this section, we discuss strategies to maximize the effectiveness of such communication.

The majority of research about communication of life-limiting prognosis and discussions of goals of care has taken place within the construct of palliative care. For this reason, similar constructs will be utilized when we discuss effective concepts and phrases to foster communication. These elements should serve as a general guide for clinicians. Above all, physicians should tailor their approach for communication to individual patient and family decision-making preferences.

Special considerations need to be taken into account when communicating with older patients. Issues such as hearing loss, visual impairment, dementia, and delirium can impact the effectiveness of communication. Furthermore, because of an acute or chronic condition (i.e., delirium or dementia), a surrogate decision-maker is common. Decisions regarding goals of care can involve not only the goals of the patient, but often those of multiple family members. For this reason, this section is structured around the planning and implementation of a family meeting during which prognosis and goals of care are discussed.

FAMILY MEETING: BEFORE YOU BEGIN

When planning any family meeting or when anticipating a serious or prolonged conversation, we encourage the hospitalist to follow a few basic steps to create an environment conducive to a meaningful discussion. These include finding a quiet space with enough room for all participants (patient, family members, and other health care providers) to sit comfortably. Pagers and other electronic devices should be turned off or silenced. Ensure that other key members of the patient's care team (e.g., oncologists and transplant physicians) are present if specific questions about treatment options are anticipated. The nature of hospitalist medicine is such that a long-term therapeutic relationship is unusual; if there is another healthcare provider (a primary care provider for instance) with whom the patient identifies such a relationship, it is often useful to include them in the conversation. Finally, ensure that key family members and other decision-makers are present. If needed, arrange for individuals to be present by phone.

If multiple care providers will be present for a family meeting, it is often helpful to meet ahead of time, before the patient or family is present, to discuss the goals of the meeting and identify who should be the primary speaker. Review the patient's medical history beforehand, as well as previous experiences with the patient and family members and identify any issues that could affect communication or decision-making, such as challenging family dynamics or cultural or psychosocial factors. Such measures are undertaken with the goal of providing clear, consistent communication to the patient and family.

FAMILY MEETING: THE OPENING

At the start of the meeting, have everyone introduce themselves and explain their relationship to the patient. Review the reasons for the meeting with the patient and family. Typically, a good starting point is to have the patient or family member describe in their own words his/her understanding of the patient's overall disease state and prognosis. This helps identify misunderstandings or misconceptions and allows an opportunity for clarification. Throughout the meeting, encourage the patient and family to talk and ask questions.

Many guides to communication recommend asking the patient and family how they prefer to receive information. This is designed to identify if patients would benefit from visual depictions (e.g., being shown a mass on imaging) or printed materials (e.g., patient education materials) to aid in communication. Use this time to clarify how much the patient wants to know about their disease and prognosis.

FAMILY MEETING: ELEMENTS OF EFFECTIVE COMMUNICATION

Common components of goals-of-care discussions are included in Table 5.5, which is adapted from a series of articles originally published the *Journal of the American Medical Association*, now updated and collated into a book, entitled, "Care at the Close of Life: Evidence and Experience" [10]. These points should be applied to patient communication at all times, but are especially important when discussing aspects of prognosis and planning for care at the end of life.

Depending on the nature of the conversation, the clinician should be prepared for a variety of responses, from disbelief to anger to fear. Recognize that all are common grief reactions. Do not argue or contradict; instead, it can be helpful to identify and validate the emotion being expressed. Depending on the scenario, asking the patient or family member to elaborate on his/her response may provide a window into the individual's hopes and concerns.

Uncertainty is a common factor in almost every medical decision, and acknowledgment of such is important. Physicians can help manage uncertainty by ensuring that the patient has all the information needed to make difficult decisions, and by providing his/her professional recommendation. Such recommendations should be based on careful consideration of the patient's clinical scenario and their goals of care. Often, effective communication first entails articulating a shared understanding of the patient's "goals

TABLE 5.5   Components of Effective Communication[a]

Establish trust/encourage families to talk

"Tell me what you understand of your illness."

"I'm sure this illness has been a lot to absorb quickly. How are you coping with this?

"You just mentioned being scared. Can you tell me more about what scares you most?"

Respect

"I'm impressed that with everything you've gone through, you're thinking of your family."

"I can tell that through all of this, you've been a strong advocate for your father."

Support

"I want to reassure you that no matter what the road holds ahead, we will continue to offer the best care we can to ensure your comfort."

Hope

"I know that you are hoping your disease will be cured. Are there other things you want to focus on?"

"I wish, too, that this disease would stay in remission. If we cannot make that happen, what other goals might we work towards?"

Attend to affect

"Is talking about these issues difficult for you?"

"Of course talking about this makes you feel sad. It wouldn't be normal if it didn't."

[a]Adapted from McPhee SJ, Winker MA, Rabow MW, Pantilat SZ, Markowitz AJ. *Care at the Close of Life: Evidence and Experience.* New York: McGraw-Hill, 2011 [10].

of care." In order to be able to make effective care recommendations, one needs to be able to guide the patient (or family or surrogate decision-maker) in their efforts to articulate these wishes. A useful way to frame this discussion is to have the patient or family try to envision short-term and longer-term goals. The provider can then consider medical interventions and treatments as having potential benefit if these are able to help the patient meet these goals without adding additional risk or burden to the patient. Some examples of individualized patient goals could include the following:

- A desire to be alive for a certain event in the near future (e.g., the birth of a grandchild and an upcoming graduation or wedding)
- A desire to achieve or maintain a certain amount of functional ability so as to remain as independent as possible for quality of life reasons
- A goal for pain or other symptom control

- A preference for a one's death to occur in a specific place or with loved ones around (e.g., at home, or alternatively, not at home so as not be burdensome to family).

Often, we are communicating directly with surrogates and delineating a plan based on the surrogate's knowledge of the patient's wishes or values. Only when a patient's individual goals and wishes are understood can realistic, manageable, and appropriate recommendations be rendered that match the patient's preferences. Recommendations often include those addressing code status (addressed in detail below), life-sustaining treatments such as dialysis, and those addressing optimal place and type of care, including hospice services, if appropriate.

FAMILY MEETING: CLOSING AND FOLLOW-UP

As the family meeting reaches its end, the person leading the meeting should review the discussion and the decisions reached. Any points that require follow-up should also be reviewed (e.g., questions for a subspecialist who was not present); when possible, the people responsible for each follow-up issue should be identified. Finally, a plan should be made for future communication, so that the patient and family understand that the avenues of communication will be kept open.

The clinician should be prepared for the common occurrence that the "big" decisions may be deferred. Often times, the patient and family wish to discuss major medical decisions among themselves to reach a consensus. Other times, additional time may be needed to allow for the grief that can come from a new diagnosis or other bad news. In these situations, it is important to allow the patient and family adequate time to process information before pressing for a decision.

GOALS OF CARE: SPECIFIC TOPICS AND SCENARIOS

Code Status and Do-Not-Resuscitate Orders

Among patients and clinicians, a great deal of confusion exists regarding a do-not-resuscitate (DNR) order. Strictly speaking, a DNR order only refers to the care received in the event of a cardiopulmonary arrest, and does not represent an overall deescalation of care. Patients with a DNR order in place can still be hospitalized and receive ICU-level care, including the use of vasopressors and broad-spectrum antimicrobials; can still undergo elective intubation for surgical procedures; and can still receive nonurgent cardioversion (e.g., for stable atrial fibrillation).

Discussion of code status is often the first time that patients and families are confronted with limitations of aggressive care. As such, code status decisions are often difficult. In addition to the elements of effective communication mentioned above, there are several conversational techniques that the clinician can implement to provide a useful framework to this challenging discussion [11]. First, it is important that the patient understands what exactly is under discussion. The specific meaning of a DNR order should be discussed. Again, patients may be under the false impression that a DNR order is tantamount to enrollment in hospice care. In a similar vein, many clinicians find it helpful to discuss the process of a cardiopulmonary resuscitation. Using layman's terms, a description of chest compressions, electric cardioversion, and intubation can help the patient understand the frankly violent procedures related to a cardiopulmonary arrest.

Second, the clinician should feel comfortable conveying, in broad terms, what a cardiopulmonary arrest would mean to a patient's outcome. Overall, the chance of surviving an in-hospital cardiac arrest is 40%, and the chance of surviving to hospital discharge is 13%. The chance of surviving a cardiac arrest goes down dramatically in certain populations, including those >65 years of age, those on dialysis, or those with metastatic cancer [12]. Thus, for the majority of patients, a cardiac arrest represents an end of life event characterized by painful invasive procedures. This is in stark contrast to cardiac arrests as portrayed on television and in movies, where almost 70% of such scenarios result in a rapid and full recovery with little evidence of residual neurological impairment.

Finally, the decision regarding code status should be placed in the larger context of a patient's goals of care. As mentioned above, the clinician should not shy away from making a recommendation based on his/her knowledge of the patient's disease process and the patient's expressed goals. If a patient identifies independence, being able to interact with loved ones, or dying at home as important goals, the physician should feel comfortable recommending a DNR order in the presence of a limited prognosis.

The Role of Advance Directives in Decision-Making

Advance directives are documents that detail a person's wishes with respect to life-sustaining treatment (typically called a living will) and their choice for surrogate decision-maker (typically called a durable power of attorney for health care). These documents were first developed in the 1970s with the goal of protecting a patient's autonomy and reducing the perceived disparity between a patient's goals of care and the care received at the end of life. Currently, all Medicare-certified institutions are required by federal law to provide patients with information regarding their right to formulate advance directives, and a recent survey found that up to 70% of community-dwelling older adults have completed an advance directive. Recent studies have shown that the presence of an advance directive increases that chance that the care a patient receives is in concordance with their preferences. In geriatric populations, these documents are especially important, as an estimated 70% of elderly Americans lack decision-making capacity at the end of life [13].

For hospitalists, the presence of an advance directive can help guide surrogate decision-makers in the use of the principle of substituted judgment, which attempts to answer the question of what the patient would want if he or she were able to participate in the decision-making. In the course of discussing goals-of-care for a patient that lacks decision-making capacity, the goals expressed within an advanced directive should always be given significant consideration, and appropriate efforts should be made to respect the goals expressed within.

Dealing with Conflict: The Family That Wants "Everything" and the Concept of Futile Care

A difficult scenario that healthcare providers encounter is the patient or the family that wants "everything" done despite an apparent poor prognosis. Often times, this request is interpreted as the desire to have everything and anything done to extend life, no matter how invasive or how low the likelihood of success. Although infrequent in number, these situations can be the cause of significant moral distress among care providers, who describe frustration or grief at providing seemingly "futile" care at the end of life.

The angst caused by these situations is reflected in the body of literature that exists around these scenarios, and several recent reviews describe approaches to this difficult situation [14]. At the core of these reviews are the general principles of effective communication mentioned earlier, including a careful exploration of the goals, values, and beliefs that underlie these requests. Such an evaluation can reveal, for example, misunderstandings of the disease leading to unrealistic expectations; the fear that limitations to care mean "giving up"; or a faith-based belief that all efforts should be made to extend life. After this initial exploration, the clinician can address any specific concerns with the help of other care providers as indicated (subspecialists to address questions of disease-related prognosis or members of a chaplain service to address religious concerns) and recommend an approach to treatment that captures the patient's values and goals. In the event that significant conflict among decision-makers and the healthcare team remain despite efforts at reaching common ground, it is important that the hospitalist consider bringing other resources to the discussion. Many hospitals have a means by which patient–doctor conflict can be resolved, which may include a formal ethics or palliative care consultation.

A common concept that is often raised in this situation is that of medical futility, loosely defined as a plan of care that either has no pathophysiological rationale or would serve no meaningful purpose to the patient. This idea is often raised when a patient or family is requesting care that the clinician considers of limited or no value. While it is true that healthcare providers are under no obligation to perform or offer care that is of no medical benefit, we urge caution in applying this notion broadly to doctor/decision-maker conflict. A study of medically futile situations brought before the legal system revealed that even among specialists, a great deal of disagreement exists regarding what therapies are considered "futile" in a variety of medical scenarios. Thus, futility as a means by which a patient's or family's decision are overridden should be used with extreme caution [15]. Again, in these situations, an ethics consult can provide guidance to the provider.

With the development and refinement of medical technologies, increasingly new interventions are brought to bear to both extend and improve the quality of life. When the decision is made to limit aggressive care, patients and families often wrestle with specific aspects of care, including when to stop dialysis; when to deactivate an automatic implantable cardioverter-defibrillator or pacemaker; or when to stop artificial nutrition or hydration. Rather than detail the approach to each specific situation, we wish to make the hospitalists aware that for most specific therapies in question, literature exists that can guide the decision-making process. In general, though, each intervention should be evaluated with the question: "Does this therapy/medication/device bring the patient closer to or farther away from their goals of care?" It should be emphasized that if a therapy is discontinued, possible resulting symptoms should be anticipated with a plan in place for management (i.e., dyspnea if bilevel positive airway pressure is discontinued or confusion if dialysis is withdrawn). A common area of debate and conflict is that of hydration and nutrition at the end of life, particularly in patients with advanced dementia. This is discussed in detail in Chapter 8.

PLANNING FOR THE END OF LIFE: HOSPICE CARE

When a patient and/or family makes the decision to stop aggressive treatment with curative intent, the hospitalist should feel confident discussing the option of hospice care. During the past decade, the percentage of people enrolled in hospice at the time of death has increased markedly to more than

40% in 2009. Traditionally, hospice was designed to care for patients with terminal cancer, and while terminal cancer remains one of the most common conditions for which a patient is enrolled in hospice, noncancer diagnoses now make up the majority of hospice admissions in the United States.

As described above, hospice care is reserved for those patients who are not expected to live longer than 6 months and who have decided to change the goals of care from curative to comfort-based. Hospice care utilizes a patient and family-centered model of care that extends services to the family even after the patient has passed away. Hospice care involves a multidisciplinary team of doctors, nurses, social workers, home health aides and chaplains; this care can be delivered in a variety of settings, including the patient's residence, a nursing home, or a dedicated in-patient hospice facility.

When discussing hospice with a patient and family, a few points should be emphasized. First, when a patient is transitioned to hospice care, the patient's comfort becomes the primary goal. Any therapy that the patient receives (such as medications, nutritional support, and dialysis) is interpreted in this light. Often this means that the majority of intensive or invasive therapies are discontinued, including parenteral nutrition/hydration; chemotherapy/radiation, and blood transfusions. Exceptions can be made in certain cases and often vary among hospice organizations. Before discussing specifics with a family, it can be helpful to put a family in touch with a hospice representative, or call upon a social worker or member of the discharge planning team who can obtain this information from various local hospices.

Second, patients and families should be made aware that the decision to enroll in hospice can be withdrawn at any time and reinitiated at a later time. Finally, a common misconception of home hospice is that a nurse or other care provider is in the home continuously. This is not the case. At most, a hospice employee (nurse, health aide, etc.) is in the home a few hours, several times a week. The primary burden of care remains with the family and, depending on the needs of the patient, can be significant. If a patient or caregivers cannot meet the needs of the patient in the home even with hospice support, efforts should be made to find alternative placement, such as a nursing home or inpatient hospice.

Medicare and most private health insurance plans have a hospice benefit that covers the cost of hospice services. However, most insurance plans do not cover the "room and board" fee of an inpatient hospice facility, which generally ranges anywhere from $150 to $400 a day. Medicaid, on the other hand, does cover such a fee; however, patients and families may not want to "spend down" to the point where they can apply for Medicaid coverage. Though potentially difficult, patients and families need to carefully consider financial and other practical implications of enrolling in hospice care. Again, the input of team members from social work or discharge planning can be instrumental in devising a viable plan of care that includes an appropriate place of care where the patient can receive hospice services.

CONCLUSION

Compared with the general population, those over the age at 65 are more likely to be diagnosed with life-limiting conditions or suffer the end-stage effects of a chronic illness. The skill set of any clinician who takes care of this demographic must include the ability to determine and discuss prognosis, negotiate appropriate and realistic goals of care, and effectively plan for care at the end of life. Hospitalists, who are more likely to care for frail older adults during acute deteriorations in their health or during transitions from slow decline to active dying, play a fundamental role in these discussions and should develop the tools necessary to help guide their patients toward a dignified death in a location and manner of their choosing whenever possible.

REFERENCES

1. Sudore RL, Fried TR. Redefining the "planning" in advance care planning: Preparing for end-of-life decision making. *Ann Intern Med* 2010;153:256–261.
2. Zhang B, Wright AA, Huskemp HA, et al. Health care costs in the last week of life: Associations with end-of-life conversations. *Arch Intern Med* 2009;169:480–488.
3. Temel JS, Greer JA, Muzikansky A, et al. Early palliative care for patients with metastatic non-small-cell lung cancer. *N Engl J Med* 2010;363:733–742.
4. World Health Organization. Cancer pain relief and palliative care: Report of a WHO expert committee. World Health Organization Technical Report Series; 804, Geneva, Switzerland, 1990.
5. Christakis NA. *Death Foretold: Prophecy & Prognosis in Medical Care*. Chicago: University of Chicago Press, 1999.
6. Anderson F, Downing GM, Hill J. Palliative Performance Scale (PPS): A new tool. *J Palliat Care* 1996;12:5–11.
7. National Hospice Organization Standards and Accreditation Committee Medical Guidelines Task Force. Medical guidelines for determining prognosis in selected non-cancer disease. *Hosp J* 1996;11:47–63.
8. Reisberg B. Functional Assessment Staging (FAST). *Psychopharmacol Bull* 1988;24: 653–659.
9. Mitchell SL, Kiely DK, Hamel MB, et al. Estimating prognosis for nursing home residents with advanced dementia. *JAMA* 2004;291:2734–2740.
10. McPhee SJ, Winker MA, Rabow MW, Pantilat SZ, Markowitz AJ. *Care at the Close of Life: Evidence and Experience*. New York: McGraw-Hill, 2011.

11. Loertscher L, Reed DA, Bannon MP, et al. Cardiopulmonary resuscitation and do-not-resuscitate orders: A guide for clinicians. *Am J Med* 2010;123:4–9.

12. Ebell MH, Becker LA, Barry HC, et al. Survival after in-hospital cardiopulmonary resuscitation: A meta-analysis. *J Gen Intern Med* 1998;13:805–816.

13. Silveira MJ, Kim SYH, Langa KM. Advance directives and outcomes of surrogate decision making before death. *N Engl J Med* 2010;362:1211–1218.

14. Quill TE, Arnold R, Back AL. Discussing treatment preferences with patients who want "everything." *Ann Intern Med* 2009;151:345–349.

15. Lo B. *Resolving Ethical Dilemmas: A Guide for Clinicians*, 4th ed. Baltimore, MD: Lippincott, Williams & Wilkins, 2009.

CHAPTER 6

GERIATRIC PHARMACOTHERAPY

Gabe Solomon
Macgregor A. Montaño
Paul C. Walker

Older adults are living longer and taking more medications than ever before. In the United States, more than 80% of geriatric patients take a prescription drug, and approximately 40% take more than five medications [1]. As a whole, the United States spent $300 billion on pharmaceuticals in 2010 and the number of prescriptions filled by elderly patients increased dramatically with the implementation of Medicare Part D in 2003.

Increased medication use places geriatric patients at risk of unnecessary treatment and adverse drug events (ADEs), which can result in reduced quality of life, hospitalization, and even death. Geriatric patients, who often have multiple comorbidities and complex medication regimens, are four times more likely to have an adverse drug reaction (ADR) than nonelderly patients, and are more likely to be admitted to the hospital as a result [2]. Reduced organ function, loss of robust compensatory mechanisms, and decreased reserve capacity all render the elderly particularly susceptible to medication toxicity.

The goal of this chapter is to develop a framework for hospitalists to optimize medication use in older adults in the acute care setting. Overcoming challenges in prescribing for older adults, identifying inappropriate medications, and avoiding ADRs will be reviewed with an emphasis on commonly used, high-risk medications in the hospitalist's armamentarium. The chapter will address transitional care issues since older patients are particularly vulnerable to fragmented care when moving between care settings.

Hospitalists' Guide to the Care of Older Patients, Edited by Brent C. Williams, Preeti N. Malani, and David H. Wesorick.

CHALLENGES IN PRESCRIBING FOR OLDER ADULTS

A fundamental barrier to safe and effective medication use in the geriatric population is the absence of a strong evidence base to guide clinical decision-making. Study of this patient population is abundantly confounded by a lifetime of exposure to infinitely diverse variables. Disentangling the true effect of age or an active treatment from the effects of all past treatments and from years of insult by chronic and comorbid disease presents a challenge to even the most capable biostatistician.

Representation in Clinical Trials

Although geriatric patients suffer a disproportionate burden of disease and account for the most consumption of prescription drugs, they have been underrepresented in clinical trials. As a result, many studies do not provide adequate risk–benefit estimation for older adults. Medication doses recommended by premarketing trials conducted in young patients are often inappropriate for older patients [3]. Furthermore, trial design frequently fails to include measurement of adverse drug effects of greatest importance to older adults, such as falls and functional and cognitive impairment [4].

Insufficient representation occurs for multiple reasons and extends beyond practical issues like transportation, communication barriers, and physical immobility. Social factors, such as ageism, underinsurance, and economic constraints also play a role. Often, older patients are excluded because of comorbid conditions or use of a medication that interacts with the investigational treatment [5].

Hospitalists should evaluate the literature closely before assuming that results from a clinical trial are applicable to their geriatric patient. An example of how difficult and dangerous it can be to apply the findings of a trial in the general population to geriatric patients is the use of spironolactone in advanced heart failure. The Randomized Aldactone Evaluation Study (RALES) demonstrated that adding spironolactone to standard therapy in patients with severe heart failure improved outcomes [6]. In that study, 2% of patients developed hyperkalemia. An observational study of 1.3 million older adults following the publication of the RALES trial showed that older patients on combined therapy had fourfold the rate of hospital admission for hyperkalemia than those provided standard treatment. In addition, the older patients did not have the same significant decrease in rates of readmission for heart failure or death reported in the original study [7].

Trials of cancer and acute coronary syndrome treatments fall short in enrolling the population most afflicted. Patients over age 65 account for the majority of all cancer cases, but in one analysis of 16,396 cancer patients enrolled in trials, only 25% were over age 65 [8]. Though 60% of myocardial infarction deaths and the bulk of cardiac complications occur in people 75 years or older, this age group accounted for 6.7% of those enrolled in almost 600 acute coronary syndrome trials from 1966 to 2000 [9].

The U.S. Food and Drug Administration (FDA) published international industry guidelines in 1994 aimed at improving geriatric representation in Phase 3 studies [10]. The nonbinding document discourages upper age cutoffs and calls for enrollment of at least 100 subjects over age 65 in trials studying diseases that occur in but are not unique to the elderly. In diseases specific to the aged, the expectation is that the "major portion" of those enrolled would be geriatric patients. The guidance endorses the study of pharmacokinetic, dose–response, and drug–drug interactions relevant to older patients. In 1998, the FDA formally acknowledged the need for more diverse representation in clinical trials [11]. Labeling requirements were updated in 2011 to mandate dosage and administration information for special populations, including geriatric patients [12].

Altered Response to Medication

Age-related changes in pharmacokinetics and pharmacodynamics and the cumulative effect of chronic disease can influence drug response. Older adults experience important changes in the time course of drug absorption, distribution, metabolism and, most notably, elimination of medication. The action and effect of medication is also altered in the aged.

Pharmacokinetic Changes

Absorption   Most medications are absorbed in the small intestine through passive diffusion. In older patients, absorption is delayed by slowed gastric emptying and transit time through the small intestine. While the delay usually does not affect overall bioavailability, it can lead to an increased time to maximal effect. In practice, this can lead to repeated dosing of medications, such as opioid analgesics, and consequently, to increased risk of toxicity [13].

Another physiological change relevant to drug absorption is increased gastric pH [14]. Hypochlorhydria can decrease uptake of iron and calcium salts. Changes in skin and muscle in older patients can also alter absorption of medications administered topically, transdermally, or by subcutaneous or intramuscular injection.

Since older adults tend to be on multiple medications, they are at increased risk of interactions that occur because of simultaneous administration. For example, fluoroquinolone or tetracycline antimicrobials taken with calcium, magnesium, iron, or zinc containing antacids or supplements can result in clinically significant reductions in bioavailability.

Distribution   Geriatric patients have decreased total body water and lean muscle and an increased percentage of body fat [14]. These age-related changes in body composition can alter the volume of distribution of medications.

Water-soluble medications, such as aminoglycosides, have a smaller volume of distribution in older adults and generally need to be prescribed in lower doses. Other hydrophilic substances include ethanol and lithium. Medications that distribute to lean muscle, like digoxin, have smaller volumes of distribution and also warrant conservative dosing.

Lipophilic medications, on the other hand, distribute widely in older patients and may have prolonged effects as a consequence. Diazepam, for example, accumulates in the fatty tissue of older patients, resulting in slower elimination and a longer duration of action.

The extent to which a medication is bound to plasma proteins like albumin and alpha-1 acid glycoprotein also influences drug distribution. Though not a consequence of normal aging, some older adults have low albumin levels because of malnourishment or disease. Hypoalbuminemia can result in a higher fraction of the unbound (i.e., active) drug in circulation. Consequently, patients may exhibit exaggerated responses to relatively small dose adjustments of highly protein-bound drugs like phenytoin or warfarin [15]. Displacement interactions in a regimen containing multiple highly protein-bound drugs can result in dramatic changes in the free fraction, which are potentially clinically significant.

Metabolism   The liver is the primary site of drug metabolism with the lungs, intestinal walls, and kidneys playing a lesser role. Hepatic blood flow and liver size and mass are all decreased in the elderly. Reduced blood flow can result in decreased first-pass metabolism and higher bioavailability of high extraction ratio drugs, like morphine, verapamil, and propranolol.

The effect of age on the enzymatic activity of the P450 system is difficult to quantify and characterize—especially since cytochrome activity is heavily influenced by disease, concurrent medications, genetics, and lifestyle factors. In general, it is believed that the rate of medication clearance through Phase I (oxidative) metabolic pathways is unchanged or slightly reduced by aging. Phase II (conjugative) clearance is thought to be unaffected [14].

Elimination   The effects of age on the kidney are well established, and decreased renal function is the most clinically relevant change to consider when treating older adults. Glomerular filtration decreases secondary to

TABLE 6.1   Formulas for Estimating Renal Function

Cockcroft–Gault Equation:

$$\text{Creatinine Clearance (mL/min)} = \left\{ \frac{(140\text{-age in years})(\text{mass in kg})}{72 \text{ (serum creatinine in mg/dL)}} \right\} (0.85 \text{ if female})$$

Revised Abbreviated MDRD:

Estimated GFR (mL/min/1.73 m^2) = 175 (serum creatinine in mg/dL)$^{-1.154}$ (age in years)$^{-0.203}$ (0.742 if female) (1.212 if African-American)

---

diminished blood flow and a reduction in the number of functioning nephrons [16]. Moreover, renal function in the older adult is decreased by the cumulative damage of chronic diseases, like hypertension and diabetes. Of people 60–69 years of age, 7% have a glomerular filtration rate (GFR) of less than 60 mL/min/1.73 m^2. After age 69, the prevalence increases to 26% [17].

It is important to base clinical decisions on estimated GFR as opposed to serum creatinine concentration. Because of a reduction in lean muscle mass, the serum creatinine overestimates an elderly patient's kidney function. No single means of estimating renal function is well validated in the elderly [18]. The two most commonly used methods are the Cockcroft–Gault Equation (CG), which estimates creatinine clearance in a rate expressed as mL/min, and the Modification of Diet in Renal Disease (MDRD) method, which reports results per unit of body surface area, that is, mL/min/1.73 m^2. The formulas are shown in Table 6.1.

The estimates can differ in the elderly, with the MDRD generally resulting higher estimates of renal function [19]. Most clinical laboratories report estimated GFR using the MDRD method. However, because of the 1998 FDA *Guidance for Industry*, most pharmaceutical manufacturers suggest drug dose adjustments based on the CG creatinine clearance [11].

Caution is warranted in applying any equation to older adults that are underweight or obese, have compromised nutritional status, altered body composition (e.g., sarcopenia and amputation), or serum creatinines that are not at steady state. When deciding on an appropriate dose, a clinician must weigh the risk of toxicity against the risk of subtherapeutic treatment. Chemotherapy or antimicrobial dosing that fails to reach therapeutic thresholds can result in poor outcomes, prolonged treatment, and increased cost.

Pharmacodynamic Changes

There are many age-related pharmacodynamic changes that have been well characterized [14, 19]. These include changes in receptor number or affinity and altered homeostatic mechanisms.

The most clinically relevant changes occur in the cardiovascular system. Catecholamine levels increase with age, and the subsequent downregulation of beta adrenergic receptors leads to the blunting of effects of beta blockers and beta agonists [20]. Older patients are more sensitive to QT-prolonging medications, which can increase the risk for torsades de pointes. The aged also exhibit a diminished capacity for baroreceptors to sense and respond to postural changes. Antihypertensive treatment compounds the risk of orthostatic hypotension and can have serious consequences if symptoms of dizziness result in a fall.

The central nervous system (CNS) is also altered. The brain of the older adult has a smaller reserve of neurotransmitters and a more permeable blood brain barrier than that of the young. As a result, the elderly are more sensitive to psychoactive substances, particularly benzodiazepines, opioids, and medications with anticholinergic or dopaminergic properties. Even agents thought to have minimal CNS side effects, such as second-generation antihistamines, can be problematic in older patients [21].

Pharmacodynamic and pharmacokinetic changes warrant caution and awareness when prescribing medications to older patients. The use of lower doses, longer dosing intervals, and longer periods between changes in dose should be considered. Conservative prescribing practices reduce the chance of medication intolerance and toxicity [22].

POLYPHARMACY

The most basic definition of polypharmacy refers to a patient taking multiple medications. More often, the term is used to describe excessive use of medication or the use of medication that is not clinically indicated. Patients at greatest risk of polypharmacy include older patients taking five or more drugs, those with multiple physicians and pharmacies, those with impairments in vision or dexterity, and individuals recently hospitalized [23]. As prescriptions increase, so does the risk of drug–drug interactions and the development of adverse effects that are of particular concern in the elderly, such as cognitive impairment, delirium, and falls. Finally, polypharmacy impedes medication adherence.

Although older adults represent 12.4% of the U.S. population, they account for 34% of all prescription drug spending [24]. Nearly 20% of community-dwelling adults over age 65 take 10 or more medications [25]. Use of herbal and dietary supplements by older adults is also high, with more than 49% reporting having used at least one in 2006 [26].

Following evidenced-based guidelines in geriatric patients with multiple chronic diseases can lead to polypharmacy. A 12-medication regimen is recommended for a patient with chronic obstructive pulmonary disease, type 2 diabetes, osteoporosis, hypertension, and osteoarthritis [27].

Hospitalists caring for patients also need to consider life expectancy and the expected benefit of treatment. In patients with poor functional status or at the end of life, hospitalists should align prescribing to the patient's goals of care. Often, hospitalized patients at the end of life continue to receive medications that lack short-term benefit but still contribute to adverse effects and drug interactions [28]. For example, patients with limited life expectancies should rarely be continued on bisphosphonates, statins, or other medications used for primary or secondary prevention.

Prescribing Cascades

Adverse drug reactions in the elderly often mimic the conventional image of aging. Common reactions include confusion, dizziness, fatigue, falls, and incontinence. Prescribing cascades occur when a new drug is prescribed to treat an unrecognized side effect of a medication the patient is already taking [29]. As additional medications are prescribed, the patient's risk for additional ADEs increases.

One well-documented cascade involves patients with cognitive impairment treated with cholinesterase inhibitors. Cholinesterase inhibitors like donepezil, galantamine, and rivastigmine can have cholinergic effects that manifest as diarrhea or urinary incontinence. Unrecognized, this adverse medication effect commonly triggers prescription of an anticholinergic medication targeting bladder symptoms. The resultant anticholinergic effect may lead to confusion, falls or urinary retention—and possible negation of the beneficial effects of the initial treatment [30].

Another cascade involves the development of extrapyramidal effects from treatment with antipsychotics or the gastrointestinal agent metoclopramide. This can lead to inappropriate diagnosis of Parkinson's disease. Subsequent treatment with antiparkinsonian therapy can result in orthostatic hypotension and delirium [31]. Other examples of prescribing cascades are shown in Table 6.2.

Overmedication in older adults can confound proper diagnosis and prolong the hospital length of stay. Hospitalists must work to establish an accurate diagnosis before prescribing and must resist the impulse to medicate symptoms.

Identifying Potentially Inappropriate Medications

At admission, clinicians should critically evaluate each drug for appropriate indication and dose and for potential interactions. Evidence suggests that age

TABLE 6.2 Common Prescribing Cascades

Initial treatment	Effect	Subsequent treatment
Antihypertensive	Dizziness	Meclizine
CCB	Edema	Loop diuretic
NSAID	Hypertension	Antihypertensive
Cholinesterase inhibitor	Urinary incontinence	Anticholinergic
Antipsychotic	Extrapyramidal symptoms	Antiparkinsonian treatment
Thiazide	Hyperuricemia	Gout treatment
Anticholinergic or sedative	Memory problems	Dementia treatment

CCB, calcium channel blocker; NSAID, nonsteroidal anti-inflammatory drug.

over 85 years, polypharmacy, and the number of comorbidities increase a patient's risk of suffering an ADE while hospitalized [32]. Several tools have been developed to identify potentially inappropriate medications (PIMs) [33].

The Beers Criteria

The Beers Criteria are the most well-known of the tools used to assess for inappropriate prescribing. The list was developed in 1991 by an expert panel to target inappropriate medication use in nursing home residents. The criteria were broadened to include community-dwelling elderly in 1997 and again revised in 2003. In 2012, another update was published in collaboration with the American Geriatrics Society [34].

Critics of the 2003 Beers Criteria contend the list contains medications no longer widely used, fails to consider drug–drug interactions, and does not reliably identify medications that are most likely to lead to hospitalization. Specifically, the 2003 resource does not include warnings regarding warfarin or insulin, which accounted for more than 45% of hospital admissions due to ADEs in a recent study. Beers Criteria medications were responsible for 6.6% of admissions in the study [35]. The 2012 update lists sliding scale insulin as potentially inappropriate in older adults and urges judicious use of certain antiplatelet agents and novel anticoagulants [34].

Although Beers Criteria medications may not result in admission, they can cause significant side effects in older patients admitted to the hospital. A different study of acutely ill, hospitalized geriatric patients found a third were prescribed inappropriate medications as identified by Beers and colleagues, and about half had well-recognized adverse effects of these medications [36].

Screening Tool of Older Person's Prescriptions (STOPP)

The Screening Tool of Older Person's potentially inappropriate Prescriptions (STOPP) is a recently developed method to help identify inappropriate medications that might lead to serious adverse events or hospital admission [37]. A 2011 study found that, compared to the 2003 Beers Criteria, the STOPP criteria were superior in identifying avoidable ADEs in older adults that led to hospitalization [38]. In the study of 600 patients, 66% were taking medications identified by the STOPP criteria that were considered causal or contributory to admission.

Developed in 2008 by a team of geriatricians, pharmacists, pharmacologists, and primary care physicians, the STOPP tool identifies problematic drug–drug interactions, drug–disease interactions, drugs that adversely affect older patients at risk of falls, and duplicate drug class prescriptions. The criteria are arranged by physiological system and provide an explanation as to why the medication is potentially inappropriate. Compared with the 2003 Beers Criteria, the resource is more likely to predict clinically significant adverse events and can be completed more quickly, taking approximately 3 minutes [39]. A companion tool, the Screening Tool to Alert Doctors to Right Treatment (START), cues the user to consider common prescribing omissions. The STOPP tool is available online at the following link: http://ageing.oxfordjournals.org/content/suppl/2008/10/01/afn197.DC1/afn197_suppl_data.pdf.

Other tools developed include the Improved Prescribing in the Elderly Tool (IPET) and Medication Appropriateness Index (MAI) [40, 41]. Hospitalists should review the available tools and systematically apply them to improve awareness in prescribing for geriatric patients.

Underprescribing of Appropriate Medications

Prescribing strategies that simply attempt to limit the overall number of drugs prescribed to older adults are misguided. When clinicians fail to prescribe therapies with proven benefit solely because of a patient's age, it can result in higher morbidity, mortality, and unnecessary progression of disease. Treatments for hypertension, dyslipidemia, depression, and atrial fibrillation confer clear benefit, yet these treatments are under-prescribed.

The beneficial effects of controlling hypertension in the elderly have been well substantiated. The Systolic Hypertension in the Elderly Person (SHEP) study showed that treating isolated systolic hypertension reduces stroke risk by 36% and decreases cardiovascular and all-cause mortality [42]. The Hypertension in the Very Elderly Trial (HYVET) demonstrated that reduction in blood pressure was associated with a 30% reduction in stroke, 21% decrease in death from any cause, and a 64% reduction in heart failure in patients over 80 years of age [43]. Despite strong evidence, older adults remain undertreated.

Although coronary artery disease is the most common cause of death for patients over age 65, only half of patients who have had a previous coronary event are treated with a statin for secondary prevention. A meta-analysis completed in 2008 of over 19,000 patients found that statin use was beneficial for elderly patients with coronary artery disease, with a relative risk reduction of 22% in all-cause mortality and stroke reduction of 25% [44].

Some 30% of hospitalized geriatric patients are depressed, as are an estimated 40% of patients with diagnoses of stroke, myocardial infarction, or cancer. Depression is estimated to be present in 14–42% of patients in long-term care facilities [45]. Despite evidence demonstrating antidepressants are both efficacious and well-tolerated, many older adults are reluctant to take them because of fear of dependence, stigma associated with mental illness, or a negative past experience with depression treatment [46]. The potential consequences of untreated depression are grave. While people 65 years of age and older comprise some 12% of the U.S. population, they account for 16% of suicide deaths. Though the elderly account for the lowest suicide attempt rate, they have the highest completion rate [47].

Anticoagulation in patients with atrial fibrillation is recommended to reduce the risk of stroke and is far superior to aspirin treatment. While older patients are at increased risk for bleeding, age itself is not a contraindication to antithrombotic treatment. One study in 4093 patients aged 80 years or older taking an oral vitamin K antagonist found low rates of bleeding, including fatal bleeding [48]. Fall risk is often cited as a reason to avoid anticoagulants in older adults despite a lack of support for this conclusion [49]. Other medications underutilized in geriatric patients include osteoporosis treatment and opioid analgesics for cancer pain.

ADVERSE DRUG EVENTS IN THE HOSPITAL

In 2007, the Institute of Medicine estimated that between 380,000 and 450,000 preventable ADEs occur annually in U.S. hospitals with an estimated cost of $3.5 billion [50]. ADEs comprise the single largest category of adverse event experienced by hospitalized patients and account for approximately 19% of all injuries [51]. A geriatric patient who suffers such an event is at risk for increased morbidity and mortality, prolonged hospitalization, and higher costs of care [52–54].

A meta-analysis found that the incidence of serious and fatal ADEs in hospitalized patients is extremely high. The study estimated that annually, more than 2 million hospitalized patients have serious ADEs, and more than 100,000 patients have fatal adverse events. If classified as such, they would rank between the fourth and sixth leading cause of death in the United States [55].

The most common adverse reactions are neuropsychiatric symptoms, including sedation, confusion, hallucinations, and delirium. The next most common symptoms are bleeding problems, diarrhea, and kidney failure [56]. Medication problems commonly confronting hospitalists treating geriatric patients are featured in Table 6.3, along with suggested alternatives and strategies to mitigate harm.

PRESCRIBING DURING TRANSITIONS OF CARE

Transitional care has been defined as "a set of actions designed to ensure the coordination and continuity of health care as patients transfer between different locations or different levels of care in the same location" [57]. The transition process is complex and error-prone, particularly for geriatric patients, and if poorly executed can result in fragmented, poor quality care, iatrogenic complications, and increased use of healthcare resources [58]. Medication errors, often the result of medication discrepancies, are a major cause of morbidity and mortality suffered by patients as they transition across the continuum of care [59].

Patients are at risk for medication discrepancies upon hospital admission, during transitions within the hospital (such as transfers from ICU to General Floor), and when they are discharged to home or to other settings of care. The MATCH study, which evaluated admission medication histories for errors, has shown that more than a third of patients admitted to the hospital have medication errors at admission. The study estimated that more than 11% of these errors were clinically dangerous [60]. In another study, more than 50% of elderly patients admitted from home had a medication error at admission and 38% of the errors had potential clinical implications [61].

Poor communication of medical information at transition points is responsible for as many as 50% of all medication errors in the hospital and up to 20% of ADEs [62]. Obtaining medication histories on hospital admission can be challenging, regardless of the setting from which patients are admitted. Patients and their caregivers often cannot recall all of their home medications and how these medications are taken. The regimens are often complex, consisting of multiple medications prescribed by multiple prescribers and obtained from multiple pharmacies. Low health literacy and language or cultural barriers also impact the ability of patients to communicate about their home medications. Thus, hospitalists may not have access to an accurate and complete medication list for the patient on admission.

Medication discrepancies frequently occur at hospital discharge as well. Patients admitted to the hospital frequently receive new medications

TABLE 6.3 Selected High-Risk Medications Prescribed By Hospitalists

Therapeutic class or drug	Potential harm	Comment	Strategies and alternatives
System: cardiovascular			
Amiodarone	Bradycardia, hypothyroidism, pulmonary fibrosis, ataxia, tremor, peripheral neuropathy, insomnia, impaired memory	Extremely long half life (range 25–100 days). Many significant drug interactions with commonly prescribed medication.	Generally, avoid in older patients.
Beta blockers	Diminished hypoglycemic awareness in diabetics, COPD exacerbation, bradycardia	Effect often unpredictable in older patients. May not be as efficacious as other antihypertensives in older adults without comorbidities (may increase stroke compared to others). Likely underutilized in heart failure.	Use in patients with CAD/CHF. Should not be first-line treatment for hypertension in patients without a compelling indication.
Calcium channel blockers	Constipation, edema, exacerbation of heart failure	Adverse effects are more common in the elderly but are dose dependent. Avoid treating side effects with additional medications.	Reduce dose. Choose an alternative antihypertensive.
Digoxin	Confusion, dizziness, heart block, nausea, vomiting, diarrhea, anorexia, visual disturbances	Age is a significant predictor of hospitalization for digoxin toxicity.	Lower target therapeutic range of 0.5–0.8 ng/mL provides similar benefit as higher range in older patients.
Loop diuretics	Electrolyte derangement, worsened incontinence, fall risk	Risk likely outweighs benefit when used for dependent edema. Avoid use as antihypertensive.	Exercise, elevation, compression stockings for dependent edema.

Spironolactone	Hyperkalemia	Begin with low doses, especially in individuals with decreased renal function. Monitor electrolytes closely.
System: urogenital/renal		
Alpha$_1$-blockers (terazosin, doxazosin, prazosin, tamsulosin, alfuzosin)	Dizziness, orthostatic hypotension, falls	Older patients with severe heart failure did not have decreased hospitalization and mortality seen in younger patients using this drug. One analysis showed increased risk of admission and death. Nonselective alpha blockers (doxazosin, terazosin) have greater effect on blood pressure and are more likely to result in side effects. Consider selective alpha blocker such as tamsulosin.
Antimuscarinics (oxybutynin, tolterodine, trospium, darifenacin, solifenacin, fesoterodine)	Anticholinergic effects of dry mouth, blurred vision, constipation, sedation, cognitive impairment, and urinary retention	Consider urodynamic testing to ensure that symptoms are due to overactive bladder. Check post-void residual before initiating. Favor nonpharmacological approach. Long-acting formulations better tolerated. Tolterodine least constipating and may have less distribution into the central nervous system.
System: neurologic/psychiatric		
Antihistamines, first generation (diphendydramine, hydroxyzine)	Anticholinergic effects of dry mouth, blurred vision, constipation, sedation, cognitive impairment, and urinary retention	Choose low-dose second-generation antihistamine (loratadine, cetirizine, fexofenadine), nasal saline, or nasal corticosteroid.

(*Continued*)

TABLE 6.3 (*Continued*)

Therapeutic class or drug	Potential harm	Comment	Strategies and alternatives
Antipsychotics	Cardiac arrhythmias, death (black box warning), pneumonia, metabolic effects, parkinsonism	Should be used as a last resort for behavioral symptoms of dementia.	Document risk/benefit discussion with patient/caregiver. Consider low doses of quetiapine or risperidone.
Benzodiazepines	Falls, confusion, motor vehicle accidents, cognitive impairment	Increase in fall risk may be as high as 60%.	Avoid. If necessary use lorazepam or oxazepam due to their hydrophilic properties and phase 2 metabolism. Initiate at low dose.
Tricyclic antidepressants	Anticholinergic effects of dry mouth, blurred vision, constipation, sedation, cognitive impairment, urinary retention, arrhythmia	Nortriptyline has less anticholinergic properties than amitryptyline. 2010 APA guideline recommends pretreatment electrocardiogram in patients over age 50.	Consider alternative agent.
Sedative hypnotics	Increase falls, prolonged sedation	Avoid barbiturates and benzodiazepines with long half-life or active metabolites.	Sleep hygiene. Do not recommend diphenhydramine. Use trazodone (off label use), or zolpidem for short-term management only.
System: gastrointestinal Dicyclomine, scopolamine, dimenhydrinate, meclizine, atropine, and diphenoxylate	Anticholinergic effects of dry mouth, blurred vision, constipation, sedation, cognitive impairment and urinary retention	Should be avoided in patients with BPH, glaucoma, or chronic bronchitis or emphysema.	

Diphenoxylate/atropine	Drowsiness, cognitive impairment	Because of diphenoxylates similarity to meperidine, classified as a controlled substance.
H₂ receptor antagonists (famotidine, ranitidine, cimetidine)	Central nervous effects including confusion and headache	Side effects due to accumulation in setting of decreased renal function. Tachyphylaxis with repeat dosing. Reduce dose. Treat with proton pump inhibitor.
Metoclopramide	Psychiatric symptoms (somnolence, confusion, anxiety, depression), tardive dyskinesia, and parkinsonism	
Phenothiazines (promethazine, prochlorperazine, chlorpromazine, trimethobenzamide)	Sedation, orthostatic hypotension, extrapyramidal side effects, and delirium	May also slow the rate of recovery from opiate-induced respiratory depression. Long-term use associated with increased mortality and higher level nursing care requirements. Consider ondansetron (off-label use).
Proton pump inhibitors	Rare association with pneumonia, *Clostridium difficile* infection, fracture risk, drug interactions	Concern for increase in both HAP and CAP. Increased risk of fracture may be the result of reduced calcium absorption. Consider use for protective effects in patients on anticoagulant or antiplatelet medications. Assess need for medication at time of discharge.

(*Continued*)

79

TABLE 6.3 *(Continued)*

Therapeutic class or drug	Potential harm	Comment	Strategies and alternatives
System: pulmonary			
Corticosteroids	Mood changes, edema	Complicated tapers difficult to manage and not necessary for short-term treatment.	Consider fixed-dose regimen, for example: prednisone 30–40 mg daily for 7 days.
Theophylline	Severe cardiac arrhythmias, seizures and death	Use not recommended in general. Patients over 75 years old have a 16-fold greater risk of life-threatening events or death than patients less than 25.	Inhaled or systemic corticosteroids.
System: hematology			
Aspirin	Bleeding	Lack of evidence supporting doses greater than 150 mg/day in patients age 65 or older. Lack of evidence supporting daily use of any dose in patients 80 years and older.	Consider discontinuation, especially if no coronary, cerebral or peripheral vascular disease.
Oral anticoagulants (warfarin, dabigatran, rivaroxaban)	Bleeding	May be underutilized in some geriatric patients. Dabigatran bleeding complications increased in older patients. Current guidelines do not support indefinite use in first episode of uncomplicated DVT or PE.	Adjust dabigatran dose for renal function and drug interactions. Initiate warfarin at low dose and monitor closely.

System/Drug			
System: immune			
Flouroquinolones	Tendon rupture, cardiac arrhythmias (QT prolongation), hypoglycemia, *Clostridium difficile* infection	Elevated risk of tendon rupture in older patients with concomitant corticosteroid use.	Alternative antimicrobial.
Nitrofurantoin	Pulmonary toxicity, hepatotoxicity, inadequate therapeutic concentration	Will not concentrate to effective urinary level in patients with GFR <60 mL/min.	Alternative antimicrobial.
Trimethroprim-sulfamethoxazole	Hyperkalemia, hypoglycemia, renal failure, rash	Alternatives are available which do not significantly elevate INR in patients on warfarin	Alternative antimicrobial.
System: musculoskeletal			
Opioids	Confusion, orthostatic hypotension, falls, constipation, and urinary retention	All are metabolized by the liver. Morphine has active metabolites that can accumulate in renal dysfunction. Elderly at increased risk of fatal respiratory depression with transdermal fentanyl. Risk of meperidine neurologic toxicity increased in elderly.	Reduce dose, extend dosing interval, and monitor closely. Avoid meperidine.
NSAIDs	Gastrointestinal bleeding, renal and negative cardiac effects such as worsened hypertension and heart failure		Consider scheduled acetaminophen or topical lidocaine. Consider concomitant proton pump inhibitor if NSAID use cannot be avoided.

(Continued)

81

TABLE 6.3 *(Continued)*

Therapeutic class or drug	Potential harm	Comment	Strategies and alternatives
System: endocrine			
Bisphophonates (alendronate, ibandronate, risedronate, zoledronic acid)	Nausea, heartburn, esophageal ulceration and perforation with oral therapy. Osteonecrosis of the jaw (rare).	Avoid oral therapy in patients with swallowing disorders. Be mindful of recommended renal dose adjustments.	Annual intravenous zolendronic acid for patients with esophagitis. Teriparatide or denosumab in patients who fail or cannot use bisphosphonates.
Insulin	Hypoglycemia	Consider adjusting HbA1C goal in older patients with multiple comorbidities, short prognosis or at increased risk of hypoglycemia.	Consider novel oral agents or analog insulins with less association with hypoglycemia.
Sulfonylureas	Hypoglycemia	Glyburide has an active metabolite and can result in prolonged hypoglycemia.	Glipizide does not have active metabolites.

COPD, chronic obstructive pulmonary disease; CAD, coronary artery disease; CHF, congestive heart failure; APA, American Psychological Association; HAP, hospital-acquired pneumonia; CAP, community-acquired pneumonia; NSAIDs, nonsteroidal anti-inflammatory medications; DVT, deep vein thrombosis; PE, pulmonary embolus.

or have their existing medications changed. As a result, the final list of medications at discharge may accidentally omit needed medications, duplicate existing therapies, and include incorrect dosages. One recent study found that 14% of geriatric patients recently discharged from hospital to home experienced at least one medication discrepancy within 24–72 hours of discharge [59]. Further, more patients who experienced a discrepancy were rehospitalized within 30 days of discharge because of an ADE compared with patients who did not experience a medication discrepancy. Another study documented that 59% of elderly patients experience unwanted incidents following hospital discharge; medication-related incidents were the most common type, comprising 32% of the unwanted incidents [62].

To address medication discrepancies and reduce the risk for ADEs, the Joint Commission has recommended medication reconciliation at hospital discharge as one of its patient safety goals in 2012 [63]. Despite the recommendation, however, there is little evidence to guide hospitals as to how to accomplish medication reconciliation.

The most studied method is medication reconciliation, with or without patient counseling, performed by pharmacists at discharge. Studies have had mixed results, with some finding significant reductions in hospitalization or preventable ADEs, while others have not demonstrated benefit [64–68]. One study found that a pharmacist-led intervention at the time of discharge decreased readmission rates by 16% and emergency room visits by 47%. A review showed a beneficial effect in patients with heart failure [69].

Another pharmacist intervention to consider is posthospital discharge follow-up phone calls; however, studies of this intervention have not consistently demonstrated benefit [70, 71].

Communication between the hospitalist team, patient, and outpatient team is critical. When possible, one physician should be responsible for all prescribing, and the patient should try to have their medications filled at one pharmacy. If a patient has problems with cognition, a caregiver should be instructed as well.

To provide and sustain safe, effective patient transitions between settings, the entire hospital discharge process needs to be evaluated and redesigned, with medication reconciliation being incorporated into the new process. Chapter 13 provides additional information about care transitions.

MEDICATION ADHERENCE

Assessing adherence is critical to successful medication treatment. The optimal regimen has no benefit if the patient never fills the initial prescription. Extracting accurate information about adherence requires a savvy, nonjudgmental approach. Determining the reasons for noncompliance directs strategies for improvement.

Patient Factors

Impaired hearing, vision, dexterity, cognition, and knowledge deficits contribute to suboptimal medication use in older adults. Cost and disparity between a patient or caregiver's goals of care and the healthcare provider's goals also impact adherence to treatment. Elderly patients have basic or below basic health literacy skills compared with younger patients. Hospitalists should tailor medication education to the capabilities of the individual patient.

Cost

In 2003, President George W. Bush signed the Medicare Modernization Act into law. Better known as Medicare Part D, it was designed to help cover prescription drugs for older adults who were previously without adequate prescription drug coverage. While some cost savings have been associated with Medicare Part D, out-of-pocket spending and prescription costs are still high for the elderly. Initially, patients who exceeded their coverage limit entered what was known as the "donut hole," and were required to pay all of their medication costs. Often, medication expenses would increase by hundreds of dollars per month. Approximately a quarter of seniors responded by stopping their medications because they could no longer afford them.

Under more recent healthcare law reforms, the situation has improved. Patients now receive a $250 rebate when reaching the donut hole. Once they enter the coverage gap, they qualify for a 50% manufacturer-paid discount on covered brand-name drugs. Although the patient pays half-price for the proprietary drug, the full price counts toward out-of-pocket spending and helps the senior emerge from the coverage gap. Even at a discounted rate, brand-name drug expenses can add up quickly.

Hospitalists should be aware that patients may not fill needed prescriptions if they are too expensive. Box 6.1 illustrates some strategies to reduce costs and improve compliance for patients discharged from the hospital.

Physicians and pharmacists should review medications with patients and ask about out-of-pocket costs before a patient leaves the hospital. Older patients are often grateful for such consideration and for help simplifying complicated drug regimens. Often, streamlining the medication list and setting clear expectations can engender trust in the healthcare system and improve medication safety and adherence.

BOX 6.1

MEDICATION COST-SAVING STRATEGIES

1. *Use generic alternatives.* A generic medication is a drug product that is comparable with the brand-name drug in dosage form, strength, route of administration, quality, performance characteristics, and intended use. According to the FDA, "generic drugs are identical or within an acceptable bioequivalent range to the brand-name counterpart with respect to pharmacokinetic and pharmacodynamic properties." Generic medications are up to 70% less expensive than brand-name counterparts, and pharmacists are generally allowed to substitute generic medications automatically unless a prescription is marked "Dispense as Written."

2. *Utilize therapeutic equivalents.* Many proprietary drugs do not have a generic equivalent, but often there is a therapeutically equivalent drug of the same class that is similarly effective. For example, substituting one statin medication for another.

3. *Over-the-counter equivalents.* Some prescription medicines have equivalents that can be purchased over-the-counter (OTC). Buying over-the-counter medications may save money for certain medications, such as pain medications, allergy medications, or antacids.

4. *Stop unneeded medications.* Some medications can be stopped because they are not effective, not tolerated, or are no longer needed.

5. *Avoid new "brand-only" formulations.* When a brand name drug goes off patent, the manufacturer frequently releases a new "brand-only" form that is slightly different from the original compound, often a longer-acting or single isomer formulation.

6. *Use discount prescription programs.* Many retail pharmacies offer generic prescriptions which, despite being out-of-pocket, are much cheaper than insurance copays. Commonly, 1 month will cost $4 and a 3-month supply $10. These medications do not count against the "donut hole" since they are paid for solely by the customer and not a third-party payer.

7. *Utilize low-income subsidies and prescription assistance programs.* Nearly half of Medicare beneficiaries have an income below 200% the federal poverty level, and there is a low-income subsidy for patients making less than $15,600 annually. Additionally, pharmaceutical companies have prescription assistance programs for low-income patients. Check online resources like http://rxassist.org and http://needymeds.org.

A STEP-WISE APPROACH TO PRESCRIBING FOR THE HOSPITALIZED OLDER PATIENT

Reconcile Medications

It is critical to know which medications a patient is taking at admission, transfer, and discharge. This can be difficult in older patients, especially those admitted with dementia or confusion. If the patient is unreliable, the team should attempt to verify medications by contacting family members or the patient's outpatient medical team. It is important to ask about over-the-counter medications and supplements. A good medication review is essential because discrepancies between patients' understanding of what they should be taking and what physicians record on their medication list are common. Screening for adherence is also important. Medications without indications should be discontinued.

Identify High-Risk Medications

Utilize tools such as the Beers Criteria or STOPP criteria to identify potentially inappropriate medications. Be mindful of potential drug-drug and drug-disease interactions and whether a patient's symptoms might reflect a medication side effect. Avoid prescribing cascades (see Table 6.2). If there has been a change in renal or liver function, previously prescribed medications may require dose adjustments. High-risk medications should be replaced with safer alternatives when possible. Table 6.3 provides some alternatives to commonly prescribed high-risk medications.

Consider Goals of Care

Understanding the life expectancy of patients and their goals of care can help physicians to prescribe appropriately. A short life expectancy limits the value of medications that require years to attain benefit. For patients with advanced dementia or poor functional status medications, such as statins, bisphosphonates, and cholinesterase inhibitors, are controversial. Age alone should not be a determinate in prescribing beneficial care. Patients with long life expectancy should be prescribed evidence based treatments. Medications treating coronary artery disease, hypertension, hyperlipidemia, and anticoagulation have been well studied in older patients and found effective.

Be Mindful When Starting a New Medication

Clinicians should consider the complex pharmacokinetic and pharmacodynamic changes associated with older patients. The adage "start low and go slow" is important to keep in mind, with special attention paid to medications that depend on renal clearance. Medications should be prescribed as a therapeutic trial and should be stopped or titrated if not providing the desired effect. Whenever possible use nonpharmacological approaches to combat common problems, including insomnia, incontinence, delirium, or behavior problems in patients with dementia. Consider the additive effect of medications. The impact of a new, seemingly benign medication can result in harm when added to a regimen that already contains anticholinergic, serotonergic, or dopaminergic medications.

Improve Adherence

To improve adherence, clinicians need to focus on cost, regimen, and health literacy. Patients should be asked about their ability to afford medications prior to discharge. The Box 6.1 outlines strategies to reduce cost and improve compliance for patients discharged from the hospital. Make an effort to discontinue unnecessary or marginally effective medications, use single daily dosing, and schedule medications at the same time of day. In patients with poor health literacy, interventions such as medication organizers and an educational session with a pharmacist are worthwhile. Consider an occupational therapy consult to determine a patient's ability to take medications reliably in a simulated home environment.

Improve Transitions in Care

Communication between the hospitalist team, patient, and outpatient team is critical. When possible, one physician should be responsible for all prescribing, and the patient should have medications filled at one pharmacy. Explicitly clear instructions upon discharge include indication, proper dose, administration instructions, and potential side effects. Medication reconciliation should be performed at discharge, and a 48-hour postdischarge phone call may be helpful.

REFERENCES

1. Kaufman DW, Kelly JP, Rosenberg L, Anderson TE, Mitchell AA. Recent patterns of medication use in the ambulatory adult population of the United States: The Slone Survey. *JAMA* 2002;287:337–344.
2. Beijer HJ, de Blaey CJ. Hospitalizations caused by adverse drug reactions: A meta-analysis of observational studies. *Pharm World Sci* 2002;24:46–54.
3. Cho S, Lau SW, Tandon V, Kumi K, Pfuma E, Abernathy DR. Geriatric drug evaluation: Where are we now and where should we be in the future? *Arch Intern Med* 2011;171: 937–940.

4. Halter JB, Ouslander JG, Tinetti ME, Studenski S, High KP, Asthana S. *Hazzard's Geriatric Medicine and Gerontology*, 6th ed. New York: McGraw Hill Medical, 2009.

5. Herrera AP, Snipes SA, King DW, Torres-Vigil I, Goldberg DS, Weinberg AD. Disparate inclusion of older adults in clinical trials: Priorities and opportunities for policy and practice change. *Am J Public Health* 2010;100:105–112.

6. Pitt B, Zannad F, Remme WJ, Cody R, Castaigne A, Perez A, et al. The effect of spironolactone on morbidity and mortality in patients with severe heart failure. *N Engl J Med* 1999;341:709–717.

7. Beizer JL. Rates of hyperkalemia after publication of the Randomized Aldactone Evaluation Study. *Consult Pharm* 2005;20:148–149.

8. Hutchins LF, Unger JM, Crowley JJ, Coltman CA, Jr., Albain KS. Underrepresentation of patients 65 years of age or older in cancer-treatment trials. *N Engl J Med* 1999;341: 2061–2067.

9. Lee PY, Alexander KP, Hammill BG, Pasquali SK, Peterson ED. Representation of elderly persons and women in published randomized trials of acute coronary syndromes. *JAMA* 2001;286:708–713.

10. Food and Drug Administration. Guideline for Industry: Studies in Support of Special Populations: Geriatrics. Rockville, MD, US Department of Health and Human Services. *Fed Regist* 1994;59:39398–39400.

11. Food and Drug Administration. Guidance for Industry: Pharmacokinetics in Patients With Impaired Renal Function-Study Design, Data Analysis, and Impact on Dosing and Labeling. Rockville, MD, US Department of Health and Human Services. *Fed Regist* 1998;63:6855–6860.

12. Food and Drug Administration. Guidance for Industry on Postmarketing Studies and Clinical Trials—Implementation of Section 505(o)(3) of the Federal Food, Drug, and Cosmetic Act. Rockville, MD, US Department of Health and Human Services. *Fed Regist* 2011;76:18226–18227.

13. Hammerlein A, Derendorf H, Lowenthal DT. Pharmacokinetic and pharmacodynamic changes in the elderly. Clinical implications. *Clin Pharmacokinet* 1998;35:49–64.

14. DePiro JT, Talbert RL, Yee GC, Matzke GR, Wells BG, Posey LM. *Pharmacotherapy: A Pathophysiologic Approach*, 6th ed. New York: McGraw Hill Medical, 2005.

15. Grandison MK, Boudinot FD. Age-related changes in protein binding of drugs: Implications for therapy. *Clin Pharmacokinet* 2000;38:271–290.

16. Rowe JW, Andres R, Tobin JD, Norris AH, Shock NW. The effect of age on creatinine clearance in men: A cross-sectional and longitudinal study. *J Gerontol* 1976;31:155–163.

17. National Kidney Foundation. K/DOQI clinical practice guidelines for chronic kidney disease: Evaluation, classification, and stratification. *Am J Kidney Dis* 2002;39:S1–S266.

18. Van Pottelbergh G, Van Heden L, Mathei C, Degryse J. Methods to evaluate renal function in elderly patients: A systematic literature review. *Age Ageing* 2010;39:542–548.

19. Laroche ML, Charmes JP, Marcheix A, Bouthier F, Merle L. Estimation of glomerular filtration rate in the elderly: Cockcroft-Gault formula versus modification of diet in renal disease formula. *Pharmacotherapy* 2006;26:1041–1046.

20. Pugh KG, Wei JY. Clinical implications of physiological changes in the aging heart. *Drugs Aging* 2001;18:263–276.

21. Feely J, Coakley D. Altered pharmacodynamics in the elderly. *Clin Geriatr Med* 1990;6: 269–283.

22. Hutchison LC, Sleeper RB. Battaglia DA (ed.), *Fundamentals of geriatric pharmacotherapy: An evidenced based approach*, 1st ed. Bethesda, MD: American Society of Health-System Pharmacists, 2010.

23. Mackinnon NJ, Hepler CD. Indicators of preventable drug-related morbidity in older adults 2. Use within a managed care organization. *J Manag Care Pharm* 2003;9: 134–141.

24. Stuart B, Shea D, Briesacher B. Dynamics in drug coverage of Medicare beneficiaries: Finders, losers, switchers. *Health Aff* 2001;20:86–99.

25. Steinman MA, Hanlon JT. Managing medications in clinically complex elders: "There's got to be a happy medium." *JAMA* 2010;304:1592–1601.

26. Qato DM, Alexander GC, Conti RM, Johnson M, Schumm P, Lindau ST. Use of prescription and over-the-counter medications and dietary supplements among older adults in the United States. *JAMA* 2008;300:2867–2878.

27. Boyd CM, Darer J, Boult C, Fried LP, Boult L, Wu AW. Clinical practice guidelines and quality of care for older patients with multiple comorbid diseases: Implications for pay for performance. *JAMA* 2005;294:716–724.

28. Holmes HM, Hayley DC, Alexander GC, Sachs GA. Reconsidering medication appropriateness for patients late in life. *Arch Intern Med* 2006;166:605–609.

29. Rochon PA, Gurwitz JH. Optimising drug treatment for elderly people: The prescribing cascade. *BMJ* 1997;315:1096–1099.

30. Gill SS, Mamdani M, Naglie G, Streiner DL, Bronskill SE, Kopp A, et al. A prescribing cascade involving cholinesterase inhibitors and anticholinergic drugs. *Arch Intern Med* 2005;165:808–813.

31. Rochon PA, Stukel TA, Sykora K, Gill S, Garfinkel S, Anderson GM, et al. Atypical antipsychotics and parkinsonism. *Arch Intern Med* 2005;165:1882–1888.

32. Page RL, 2nd., Ruscin JM. The risk of adverse drug events and hospital-related morbidity and mortality among older adults with potentially inappropriate medication use. *Am J Geriatr Pharmacother* 2006;4:297–305.

33. Page RL, 2nd., Linnebur SA, Bryant LL, Ruscin JM. Inappropriate prescribing in the hospitalized elderly patient: Defining the problem, evaluation tools, and possible solutions. *Clin Interv Aging* 2010;5:75–87.

34. American Geriatrics Society 2012 Beers Criteria Update Expert Panel. American Geriatrics Society updated Beers Criteria for potentially inappropriate medication use in older adults. *J Am Geriatr Soc* 2012;60:616–631.

35. Budnitz DS, Lovegrove MC, Shehab N, Richards CL. Emergency hospitalizations for adverse drug events in older Americans. *N Engl J Med* 2011;365:2002–2012.

36. Gallagher PF, Barry PJ, Ryan C, Hartigan I, O'Mahony D. Inappropriate prescribing in an acutely ill population of elderly patients as determined by Beers' criteria. *Age Ageing* 2008;37:96–101.

37. Gallagher PF, Ryan C, Byrne S, Kennedy J, O'Mahony D. STOPP (Screening Tool of Older Person's Prescriptions) and START (Screening Tool to Alert doctor to Right Treatment). Consensus validation. *Int J Clin Pharmacol Ther* 2008;46:72–83.

38. Gallagher P, O'Mahony D. STOPP [screening tool of older persons' potentially inappropriate prescriptions]: Application to acutely ill elderly patients and comparison with Beers' criteria. *Age Ageing* 2008;37:673–679.

39. Hamilton H, Gallagher P, Ryan C, Byrne S, O'Mahony D. Potentially inappropriate medications defined by STOPP criteria and the risk of adverse drug events in older hospitalized patients. *Arch Intern Med* 2011;171:1013–1019.

40. Barry PJ, O'Keefe N, O'Connor KA, O'Mahony D. Inappropriate prescribing in the elderly: A comparison of the Beers criteria and the improved prescribing in the elderly tool [IPET] in acutely ill elderly hospitalized patients. *J Clini Pharm Ther* 2006;31: 617–626.

41. Fitzgerald LS, Hanlon JT, Shelton PS, Landsman PB, Schmader KE, Pulliam CC, et al. Reliability of a modified medication appropriateness index in ambulatory older persons. *Ann Pharmacother* 1997;31:543–548.

42. SHEP Cooperative Research Group. Prevention of stroke by antihypertensive drug treatment in older persons with isolated systolic hypertension. Final results of the Systolic Hypertension in the Elderly Program [SHEP]. *JAMA* 1991;265:3255–3264.

43. Beckett NS, Peters R, Fletcher AE, Staessen JA, Liu L, Dumitrascu D, et al. Treatment of hypertension in patients 80 years of age or older. *N Engl J Med* 2008;358:1887–1898.

44. Afilalo J, Duque G, Steele R, Jukema JW, de Craen AJ, Eisenberg MJ. Statins for secondary prevention in elderly patients: A hierarchical Bayesian meta-analysis. *J Am Coll Cardiol* 2008;51:37–45.

45. Koenig HG, Blazer DG. Epidemiology of geriatric affective disorders. *Clin Geriatr Med* 1992;8:235–251.

46. Givens JL, Datto CJ, Ruckdeschel K, Knott K, Zubritsky C, Oslin DW, et al. Older patients' aversion to antidepressants: A qualitative study. *J Gen Intern Med* 2006;21: 146–151.

47. Centers for Disease Control and Prevention. National suicide statistics at a glance 2009. 2012. Available at: http://www.cdc.gov/violenceprevention/suicide/statistics/aag.html (accessed April 11, 2013).

48. Poli D, Antonucci E, Testa S, Tosetto A, Ageno W, Palareti G, et al. Bleeding risk in very old patients on vitamin K antagonist treatment: Results of a prospective collaborative study on elderly patients followed by Italian Centres for Anticoagulation. *Circulation* 2011;124:824–829.

49. Man-Son-Hing M, Nichol G, Lau A, Laupacis A. Choosing antithrombotic therapy for elderly patients with atrial fibrillation who are at risk for falls. *Arch Intern Med* 1999; 159:677–685.

50. Aspden P, Wolcott JA, Bootman JL, Cronenwett LR. *Preventing Medication Errors: Quality Chasm Series*. Washington, DC: The National Academic Press, 2007.

51. Leape LL, Brennan TA, Laird N, Lawthers AG, Localio AR, Barnes BA, et al. The nature of adverse events in hospitalized patients. Results of the Harvard Medical Practice Study II. *N Engl J Med* 1991;324:377–384.

52. Raschetti R, MennitiIppolito F, Morgutti M, Belisari A, Rossignoli A. Adverse drug events in hospitalized patients. *JAMA* 1997;277:1351–1352.

53. Classen DC, Pestotnik SL, Evans RS, Lloyd JF, Burke JP. Adverse drug events in hospitalized patients. Excess length of stay, extra costs, and attributable mortality. *JAMA* 1997;277:301–306.

54. Bates DW, Spell N, Cullen DJ, Burdick E, Laird N, Petersen LA, et al. The costs of adverse drug events in hospitalized patients. Adverse Drug Events Prevention Study Group. *JAMA* 1997;277:307–311.

55. Lazarou J, Pomeranz BH, Corey PN. Incidence of adverse drug reactions in hospitalized patients: A meta-analysis of prospective studies. *JAMA* 1998;279:1200–1205.

56. Gurwitz JH, Field TS, Judge J, Rochon P, Harrold LR, Cadoret C, et al. The incidence of adverse drug events in two large academic long-term care facilities. *Am J Med* 2005;118:251–258.

57. Coleman EA, Boult C, American Geriatrics Society Health Care Systems,Committee. Improving the quality of transitional care for persons with complex care needs. *J Am Geriatr Soc* 2003;51:556–557.

58. Coleman EA. Falling through the cracks: Challenges and opportunities for improving transitional care for persons with continuous complex care needs. *J Am Geriatr Soc* 2003;51:549–555.

59. Coleman EA, Smith JD, Raha D, Min SJ. Posthospital medication discrepancies: Prevalence and contributing factors. *Arch Intern Med* 2005;165:1842–1847.

60. Gleason KM, McDaniel MR, Feinglass J, Baker DW, Lindquist L, Liss D, et al. Results of the Medications at Transitions and Clinical Handoffs [MATCH] study: An analysis of medication reconciliation errors and risk factors at hospital admission. *J Gen Intern Med* 2010;25:441–447.

61. Cornish PL, Knowles SR, Marchesano R, Tam V, Shadowitz S, Juurlink DN, et al. Unintended medication discrepancies at the time of hospital admission. *Arch Intern Med* 2005;165:424–429.

62. Mesteig M, Helbostad JL, Sletvold O, Rosstad T, Saltvedt I. Unwanted incidents during transition of geriatric patients from hospital to home: A prospective observational study. *BMC Health Serv Res* 2010;10:1.

63. The Joint Commission. National Patient Safety Goals Effective January 1, 2012. 2011. http://www.jointcommission.org/assets/1/6/NPSG_Chapter_Jan2012_HAP.pdf (accessed April 11, 2013).

64. Al-Rashed SA, Wright DJ, Roebuck N, Sunter W, Chrystyn H. The value of inpatient pharmaceutical counselling to elderly patients prior to discharge. *Br J Clin Pharmacol* 2002;54:657–664.

65. Gillespie U, Alassaad A, Henrohn D, Garmo H, Hammarlund-Udenaes M, Toss H, et al. A comprehensive pharmacist intervention to reduce morbidity in patients 80 years or older: A randomized controlled trial. *Arch Intern Med* 2009;169:894–900.

66. Nazareth I, Burton A, Shulman S, Smith P, Haines A. Tierall H. A pharmacy discharge plan for hospitalized elderly patients—A randomized controlled trial. *Age Ageing* 2001; 30:33–40.

67. Lipton HL, Bird JA. The impact of clinical pharmacists' consultations on geriatric patients' compliance and medical care use: A randomized controlled trial. *Gerontologist* 1994;34:307–315.

68. Schnipper JL, Kirwin JL, Cotugno MC, Wahlstrom SA, Brown BA, Tarvin E, et al. Role of pharmacist counseling in preventing adverse drug events after hospitalization. *Arch Intern Med* 2006;166:565–571.

69. Koshman SL, Charrois TL, Simpson SH, McAlister FA, Tsuyuki RT. Pharmacist care of patients with heart failure: A systematic review of randomized trials. *Arch Intern Med* 2008;168:687–694.

70. Dudas V, Bookwalter T, Kerr KM, Pantilat SZ. The impact of follow-up telephone calls to patients after hospitalization. *Dis Mon* 2002;48:239–248.

71. Walker PC, Bernstein SJ, Jones JN, Piersma J, Kim HW, Regal RE, et al. Impact of a pharmacist-facilitated hospital discharge program: A quasi-experimental study. *Arch Intern Med* 2009;169:2003–2010.

CHAPTER 7

MANAGING BEHAVIORAL DISTURBANCES WITH PSYCHOACTIVE MEDICATIONS: DOS, DON'TS, AND MAYBES

David C. Belmonte
Jolene Bostwick
Amy B. Rosinski

CASE STUDY PART I

Mrs. SH is a 78-year-old married retired secretary with a 1-year history of Parkinson's disease. Her neurologist has been prescribing low dose carbidopa/levadopa to treat tremor and bradykinesia. She does not take any psychotropic medication, and her only other medication is lisinopril for hypertension. At her last neurology appointment, her Mini Mental State Examination score was 21/30, and it had been stable over the last year. She lives with her husband in an assisted-living facility, and she does most of her ADLs independently, but requires assistance with IADLs.

Her dose of carbidopa/levodopa was increased 2 weeks ago to address worsening tremor. Around the same time, she was also prescribed oxybutynin for urge incontinence by her primary care physician. In the last week, her husband reported that she developed worsening sleep disturbance and increased irritability. She has been accusing him of infidelity. Occasionally, he has observed her talking to herself and picking at the air. He brought her to the emergency room because earlier this morning, she was argumentative and combative. She accused him of plotting to get rid of her so that he could be with his mistress, and could not be consoled.

On initial evaluation in the ED, Mrs. SH was oriented to self only, exhibited impaired attention, and had fluctuating level of consciousness. A mini mental status exam could not be completed because of her inability to participate in the interview. Vital signs are normal, and physical exam is benign, other than some dyskinesia. A complete blood count, liver function tests, and renal function were obtained in the emergency room. The only notable finding was a slightly elevated white blood cell

Hospitalists' Guide to the Care of Older Patients, Edited by Brent C. Williams, Preeti N. Malani, and David H. Wesorick.
© 2013 by John Wiley & Sons, Inc. Published 2013 by John Wiley & Sons, Inc.

count of 12.1. Urinalysis is positive for leukocyte esterase and nitrites, with culture pending.

Mrs. SH remained highly agitated in the ED, striking out at nurses, and trying to get out of bed. She received haloperidol 5 mg intramuscularly, was placed in soft restraints, and admitted to the medical service.

INTRODUCTION

Psychotropic medications are generally prescribed to elderly patients in the hospital setting to address a wide array of behavioral disturbances. These can range from the withdrawn patient refusing care (e.g., refusing to eat), to the paranoid patient who believes the staff is trying to poison her with medications and strikes out at staff attempting to defend herself. Frequently, the underlying cause is difficult to determine, and is often multifactorial in origin. Many behaviors encountered during hospitalization of an elderly patient represent sequelae of delirium and dementia. This chapter will provide some guidelines for the clinician dealing with difficult behaviors encountered in the hospital and provide suggestions for medications for treating these behaviors.

ASSESSING BEHAVIORAL DISTURBANCES

The first step in addressing behavioral problems is to characterize the disturbance, attempting to be as specific as possible (Table 7.1). Commonly, staff members may report, "Mr. L. was agitated last night." The terms, "agitated" and "agitation" are too general to be helpful. It would be more useful to elicit an exact description of what the patient was directly observed to be doing. The patient may have been unable to sleep, and tossed and turned in bed throughout the night. On the other extreme, the patient may have attempted to punch the bedside nurse when he came to adjust the IV pump in the middle of the night. Both of these examples of "agitation" would presumably lead to different interventions.

In further characterizing the behavior, it is informative to understand the approximate time of onset (i.e., acute to subacute, vs. chronic). If the timeframe for the behaviors is a recent change (i.e., hours to days), delirium is likely. Behaviors that are more chronic in nature may be due to a manifestation of a preexisting primary psychiatric or medical condition. Furthermore, the clinician should determine if there is a pattern to the behaviors, such as preceding triggers or specific times of day when the behaviors occur. Since the patient may be limited in his ability to provide reliable history,

TABLE 7.1 Evaluation of Behavioral Disturbances

Characterize the disturbance	Assess the environment	Conduct comprehensive medical evaluation	Factor in pre-morbid personality feaures and coping style
• Specify behaviors • Determine time of onset • Identify triggers • Obtain collateral history	• Identify if patient is over- or understimulated • Observe inter-personal interactions • Assess for sensory deficits • Evaluate for hunger, pain, constipation, reflux • Facilitate sleep	• Review medications and reduce polypharmacy • Complete infectious workup • Rule out easily reversible conditions (TSH, B-12, Vit D) • Consider neuroimaging • Obtain EEG if seizure is susupected	• Dysthymic • Anxious • Histrionic

collateral sources, such as outpatient medical providers and family members, are useful in gathering accurate data to inform clinical decision-making.

A comprehensive medical evaluation should be completed to rule out any potentially reversible medical conditions. The most common causes include infection or an adverse reaction to medication. Be aware of the contribution of steroids, pain medications, and benzodiazepines to acute mental status change. Acute intoxication or withdrawal from substances can also cause mental status changes.

Particular attention should be paid to the anticholinergic potential of individual medications, and the total anticholinergic burden caused by the synergy of multiple medications. Blockade of acetylcholine receptor can cause worsening confusion, exacerbate delirium, and contribute to overall mental status changes [1]. A useful tool for assessing anticholinergic burden of medications can be found online from the Indianapolis Discovery Network for Dementia Anticholinergic Cognitive Burden Scale: http://www.indydiscoverynetwork.org/AnticholinergicCognitiveBurdenScale.html.

The environment should be assessed and modified to reduce overstimulation and/or understimulation. Disruptive behaviors may results from unmet needs that cannot be articulated by the patient (e.g., pain and hunger), particularly in the presence of cognitive impairment. Attempts to redirect the patient, for example, by offering food or engaging the patient with activities, can serve to distract the patient, and halt disruptive behavior. Conditions should be optimized to normalize sleep by coordinating exposure to light and keeping interruptions to a minimum. Sensory deficits may also be playing a role. Inouye et al. targeted six specific risk factors for delirium (*cognitive impairment, sleep deprivation, immobility, visual impairment, hearing impairment*, and *dehydration*) and developed standardized intervention protocols [2]. Further discussion of medical causes and common medications contributing to acute mental status changes can be found in Chapter 12.

In addition to environmental and medical factors, personality features and maladaptive styles of coping may account for some types of behaviors. All patients have engrained personality traits and differing tolerances to adversity that precedes admission to the hospital. Patients are forced to face issues of grief, loss, and mortality. The additional stress of hospitalization taxes coping skills, and personality features may become more pronounced. Some patients become demoralized and hopeless about the potential for recovery. Patients with severe anxiety pose a challenge to the provider because they may be difficult to reassure and can consume a tremendous amount of staff time. While some patients are resilient and engaged with caregivers, some individuals may become antagonistic toward the treatment team.

CASE STUDY PART 2

Ms. SH meets criteria for delirium. Her case is complex in that there are potentially multiple etiologies for an acute change in mental status, which is a common occurrence in elderly patients. Specific to this patient, there is an underlying neurological condition, and possible dementia that make her vulnerable to developing delirium. There have been recent medication changes, including the initiation of an anticholinergic agent, and an increase in a dopaminergic agent. Her urinalysis is suggestive of UTI. Furthermore, sleep deprivation also predisposes a person to developing psychosis.

While the urine culture is pending, an antibiotic may be started empirically for a presumed UTI. In the absence of clear symptoms (dysuria, urinary frequency, elevated WBC count, fever, and flank pain), some practitioners will not begin empirical therapy to avoid development of antibiotic-resistant bacterial strains. Moreover, a positive urine culture may be a sign of colonization. The dose of the carbidopa/levodopa should be decreased since this may be contributing to her psychotic symptoms. Oxybutinin should be discontinued or replaced with an agent that is less anticholinergic.

GENERAL CONSIDERATIONS FOR UTILIZING PSYCHOTROPIC MEDICATIONS TO ADDRESS BEHAVIORAL DISTURBANCES

Before prescribing medications to modify behavioral disturbances among hospitalized older patients, one must determine whether the seriousness of the behaviors actually warrants it. Physical safety is a significant concern usually factoring into this decision; the clinician must evaluate the potential that if left untreated, the behavior may lead to the harm of the patient or others. Other important considerations are whether the behavior contributes to a severe impairment of functioning or causes excessive distress to the patient. Occasionally, the clinician is pressured to act because the behavior is actually more distressing to family members and caregivers than the patient himself (e.g., disrobing).

Psychotropic medications carry formal indications as approved by the FDA for the treatment of specific recognized psychiatric illnesses. In contrast, *the use of psychotropic medication to treat behavioral disturbances is considered an off-label use.* There is limited, and sometimes equivocal evidence for efficacy for the treatment of behavior disturbances, derived primarily from case reports and studies with small sample sizes and limited controls. Some medications are associated with a significant risk of adverse effects, and may even include increased mortality. The goal is to strike a favorable balance between the risks and the potential benefit of treating the identified behavior(s).

Compared with a younger patient, significant differences exist when prescribing medication to an elderly patient. Key considerations include physiological differences associated with aging. Additionally, there is a greater likelihood that older patients have a greater number of comorbid medical conditions that may complicate selection of psychotropic medications because the agent in question may affect the medical condition and contribute to increased morbidity or even mortality. Drug–drug interactions may arise between other medications and the proposed psychiatric intervention. Elderly individuals also tend to be frailer than their younger counterparts, and may be more sensitive to side effects from psychotropic medication. For example, when prescribing to the elderly, one must be cognizant of the potential to cause falls, oversedate the patient, and worsen confusion. A general rule to follow when prescribing medication to the elderly is, "start low, and go slow."

The authors acknowledge that when behaviors become serious enough and do not respond to environmental or behavioral modification, the clinician may have little choice but to prescribe medication. A discussion with the patient and his/her advocates should occur regarding the expected effect and the potential risks associated with treatment, which should be documented in the chart. Furthermore, if a patient is prescribed a medication to address behavior in the hospital, there should be a plan in place to coordinate with outpatient providers to further monitor behaviors, evaluate for emergence for side effects and to assess the need for continuing use, and to consider discontinuing the medication if it is no longer necessary. It is not an uncommon scenario for a patient to be started on a psychoactive medication in the hospital, and to have that medication continued after discharge without an ongoing indication.

TREATMENT OF SPECIFIC BEHAVIORAL SYMPTOMS

Depression

Depressive symptoms are common in the elderly hospitalized patients, occurring in as many as 11–23% of patients in the acute hospital setting [3]. It may be characterized by the presence of low mood and/or decrease in hedonic capacity in constellation with several neurovegetative symptoms- insomnia, poor appetite, anergia, decreased concentration, psychomotor slowing. It may be difficult to distinguish whether the neurovegetative symptoms are a result of the medical illness versus major depression. In geriatric presentations of depression, patients may minimize or even deny the presence of depressed mood. It may present as increased irritability, and there may be a strong anxiety component with prominent somatic features (e.g., headache and gastrointestinal distress). When psychotic features are present, a frequent delusion is that they are functionally incapable despite having intact physical abilities.

The Geriatric Depression Scale (GDS) is a validated screen that can be given to detect depression in elderly individuals [4]. The short form of the GDS is quick and easy to administer, consisting of 15 yes/no questions pertaining to mood disturbance, and it has been translated into multiple languages. It is in the public domain, and available online via free access: http://www.chcr.brown.edu/GDS_SHORT_FORM.PDF. It also comes as an application for mobile devices.

When assessing for depression, it is important to inquire about the presence of suicidal thinking. Although rare, patients have attempted and completed suicide in the hospital setting. Elderly, white males with multiple medical comorbidities, lack of social supports, and a history of substance use carry the highest risk for suicide. If suicidal ideation is strongly suspected, a patient attendant should be assigned to monitor the patient, and a referral placed to the Psychiatry Consultation Service.

There are many antidepressants from which to select (see Table 7.2). Since there are no differences in efficacy between antidepressants, specific treatments are chosen based on their side effect profile. Moreover, there might also be financial considerations, particularly if the patient is on a fixed income. SSRIs (e.g., sertraline and escitalopram) are generally considered first-line treatment, even for a younger population, because of tolerability and cost. Furthermore, SSRIs are not fatal when taken in overdose. Citalopram

TABLE 7.2 Antidepressant Treatments

Drug or drug class		Starting dose	Maximum dose	Comments
Preferred agents	Sertraline (Zoloft)	25 mg daily	150 mg daily	• Potential for GI side effects (nausea, vomiting, and diarrhea). • Monitor for hyponatremia. • May cause platelet dysfunction.
	Escitalopram (Lexapro)	2.5 mg daily	10 mg daily	• Potential for GI side effects (nausea, vomiting, diarrhea). • Monitor for hyponatremia. • May cause platelet dysfunction. • May affect sexual function.
	Mirtazapine (Remeron)	7.5 mg QHS	30 mg QHS	• Few drug interactions. • Ideal for medically ill patients. • Stimulates appetite and causes sedation (more sedation seen with lower doses).
	Venlafaxine XR (Effexor)	37.5 mg daily	225 mg daily	• Consider if patient has not responded to SSRIs, or if wanting more activation. • Potential for GI and sexual side effects similar to SSRIs. • May cause increase in BP. • Consider with comorbid pain.
	Bupropion SR (Wellbutrin)	100 mg daily	100 mg BID	• Another agent to consider for activating effect. • Take last dose before 5 p.m. to avoid insomnia • Potential to lower seizure threshold.

(Continued)

TABLE 7.2 *(Continued)*

	Drug or drug class	Starting dose	Maximum dose	Comments
Other agents to consider	Duloxetine (Cymbalta)	20 mg daily	60 mg daily	• Avoid use if CrCl is less than 30 mL/min or those with end-stage renal disease • Avoid use in patients with heavy alcohol use or those with chronic liver disease • Consider with comorbid pain
	Nortriptyline (Pamelor)	10 mg QHS	50 mg QHS	• Consider with comorbid pain. • Still has anticholinergic properties, although better tolerated than other TCAs. • Arrhythmogenic potential, so baseline EKG recommended before starting. • Can be fatal in overdose.
Adjunctive agents	Methylphenidate (Ritalin)	2.5 mg daily	5 mg BID	• Consider in post-stroke depression or in cases of severe apathy. • Monitor BP, HR, EKG. • May cause appetite suppression.
	Triiodothyronine (Cytomel)	0.025 mg daily	0.05 mg daily	• Monitor TSH, FT4, and T3 levels.
Agents to generally avoid	Fluoxetine (Prozac)			• Long half-life. • Potential for drug interactions via Cytochrome P450 2D6.
	Paroxetine (Paxil)			• Most anticholinergic of SSRIs. • Potential for drug/drug interactions via Cytochrome P450 2D6. • Significant anticholinergic potential.
	Tricyclic antidepressants (TCAs)			• Risk for causing arrhythmias.
	Monoamine oxidase inhibitors (MAOIs)			• High potential for food/drug and drug/drug interactions. • Risk for causing hypertensive crisis, orthostatic hypotension, and anticholinergic side effects.

is no longer considered as a first choice due to recent findings of prolonged QTc interval associated with this drug. If insomnia and anorexia are the primary presenting neurovegetative features, mirtazapine is good choice because it stimulates appetite and has sedating properties. However, this would not be an ideal choice in an obese or diabetic patient. On the other hand, if the patient is lethargic, venlafaxine and bupropion tend to be more activating. Methylpenidate may also be used for augmentation in patients needing more activation. While TCAs are generally avoided due to side effects, nortriptyline is better tolerated. Duloxetine and nortriptyline are useful agents for patients with co-morbid pain and depression. Triidothyronine (T3) is another augmentation treatment. Fluoxetine, paroxetine, and MAOIs are generally avoided in the elderly population because of side effects.

Mania

In contrast to depression, mania is an elevated state of mood. Manic symptoms may be due to bipolar illness or secondary to medical condition or medication (e.g., tumor and steroids). Manic patients can present with symptoms of grandiosity, increased irritability, decreased need for sleep, rapid speech, racing thoughts, hyperkinesis, and preoccupation with goal-directed behavior.

Table 7.3 lists mood-stabilizing treatments. Anticonvulsants, antipsychotics, and lithium have been used to treat mania or labile mood states. The advantage of valproic acid is the flexibility in administration form, which can be useful if the patient is refusing oral medication. Valproic acid levels can also be measured. Olanzapine and quetiapine can be given if immediate action is necessary. Both of these agents are sedating. Olanzapine can be administered intramuscularly if necessary. With long-term use, olanzapine may contribute to the development of a metabolic syndrome. Baseline lipid panel and fasting glucose should be obtained. Also, they have the potential to prolong the QTc interval; therefore, a baseline EKG is also recommended when starting these agents. Note that IM olanzapine and lorazepam should not be administered concurrently due to incidents of mortality. Lithium is generally not recommended due to the decreased renal functioning associated with age, and the risk for serious side effects and toxicity. Carbemazepine induces Cytochrome P450 3A4, which metabolizes many drugs. In addition to being an inducer of this cytochrome, it is a substrate, and it also speeds up its own metabolism.

Anxiety

Anxiety is a subjective feeling of worry and may be associated with physical symptoms, including muscle tension, diaphoresis, gastrointestinal upset,

TABLE 7.3   Mood-Stabilizing Treatments

	Drug or drug class	Starting dose	Maximum dose	Comments
Preferred agent	Valproic acid (Depakote)	125 mg TID prn	1000 mg total daily dose (in divided doses)	• Available in regular PO, sprinkles (Depakene), and IV formulations. • Potential for causing sedation, tremor, ataxia. • Monitor for thrombocytopenia, LFT elevations. • Valproic acid levels can be measured. • Potential to raise levels of warfarin.
	Olanzapine (Zyprexa)	2.5 mg daily	15 mg daily (can be given in divided doses)	• Available in regular PO, dissolvable formulation (Zydis), and IM formulation. • Potential for orthostasis, sedation, weight gain, and other metabolic effects.
	Quetiapine (Seroquel)	25 mg BID	200 mg daily (can be given in divided doses)	• Potential for orthostasis, sedation. • Potential for orthostasis, sedation, weight gain, and other metabolic effects.
Agents to generally avoid	Lithium			• Multiple side effects (renal impairment, hypothyroidism, ataxia, tremor) and potentially lethal at toxic levels, therefore needs to be closely monitored. • Avoid NSAIDs due to potential for drug interaction. • Consult Psychiatry for consideration of this medication.
	Carbamazepine (Tegretol)			• Potential for multiple drug interactions (Cyt P450 3A4 inducer and substrate). • May cause agranulocytosis

tachycardia, and tachypnea. It may externally manifest with motor restlessness and verbal agitation. Commonly symptoms of depression and anxiety occur together. A wide variety of psychotropic classes are used to treat anxiety (refer to Table 7.4). Antidepressants (escitalopram, sertraline, and venlafaxine) are the primary medication used for anxiety. However, if the initial starting dose is high, or the dose is titrated aggressively, exacerbation of anxiety symptoms may result. Therefore, it is not unusual to initiate antidepressants at half the normal starting dose used for depression when indicated for anxiety. Bear in mind that antidepressants require some time before the anxiety improves (approximately 4–8 weeks) and patients should be informed about the delayed effect to temper expectations. Buspirone, gabapentin, and pregabalin have been used to supplement antidepressants in refractory anxiety. Sometimes, the patient's anxiety causes tremendous distress and is impairing to such a degree that immediate effect is necessary, in which case short-acting benzodiazepines are considered as a temporary treatment while waiting for the antidepressant to take effect. Benzodiazepines should be used with caution because of the potential to cause hypersomnolence, to predispose to balance problems and falls, and to cause worsening confusion. They should be avoided altogether if delirium is suspected. The atypical antipsychotic, quetiapine, can be used to alleviate anxiety in the short-term with close monitoring. Quetiapine can cause somnolence and orthostatic hypotension.

Psychosis

Psychosis is an impairment in a patient's ability to distinguish reality. It is characterized by disorganized thought process, the presence of hallucinations, and delusions. Perceptual disturbances are primarily auditory or visual in nature, but may involve tactile and olfactory hallucinations as well. The latter two hint toward a central lesion as a potential etiology. Delusions are a type of psychotic symptoms involving fixed, false beliefs that the patient may hold, contrary to cultural norms. In the elderly, psychotic symptoms may arise in the context of a mood disorder (with depression or mania), a primary thought disorder (late-onset schizophrenia), a symptom of delirium, or neuropsychiatric symptom related to dementia.

The treatment of psychosis has been through dopamine receptor (D2) blockade. Table 7.5 lists antipsychotic treatments. The newer (atypical) antipsychotics are better tolerated with regards to side effects in the elderly compared with the conventional antipsychotics. The most data have been accumulated for risperidone and olanzapine. Both come in a dissolvable form, and olanzapine has the added advantage of being available in an injectable form. Quetiapine has shown effectiveness in the treatment of psychosis in the setting of comorbid Lewy body dementia or Parkinson's because it interferes less with motor functioning from dopamine antagonism, possibly

TABLE 7.4   Antianxiety Treatments

	Drug or drug class	Starting dose	Maximum dose	Comments
Preferred agents	Escitalopram (Lexapro)	2.5 mg daily	10 mg daily	• Potential for GI side effects (nausea, vomiting, diarrhea). • Monitor for hyponatremia. • May cause platelet dysfunction. • May affect sexual function.
	Sertraline (Zoloft)	12.5 mg daily	150 mg daily	• Potential for GI side effects (nausea, vomiting, diarrhea). • Monitor for hyponatremia. • May cause platelet dysfunction. • May affect sexual function.
	Venlafaxine XR (Effexor)	37.5 mg daily	225 mg daily	• Consider if patient has not responded to SSRIs, or if wanting more activation. • Potential for GI and sexual side effects similar to SSRIs. • May cause increase in BP.
Adjunctive agents	Buspirone (Buspar)	5 mg TID	15 mg TID	• Not effective if used on an as needed basis; must be taken as scheduled
	Gabapentin (Neurontin)	100 mg TID	300 mg TID	• May cause dizziness and sedation.
	Pregabalin (Lyrica)	25 mg TID	100 mg TID	• May cause dizziness and sedation.

TABLE 7.4   *(Continued)*

	Drug or drug class	Starting dose	Maximum dose	Comments
Other agents to consider	Lorazepam (Ativan)	0.25 mg daily prn	2 mg daily (in divided doses)	• Available in PO, IM, and IV formulations. • Drug of choice in patients with liver disease. May cause somnolence, confusion. • Increased risk for falls. • Recommended for short-term use only.
	Clonazepam (Klonopin)	0.25 mg daily prn	1 mg daily (in divided doses)	• May cause somnolence, confusion. • Increased risk for falls. • Recommended for short-term use only.
	Quetiapine (Seroquel)	12.5 mg BID prn	100 mg daily (in divided doses)	• For acute, severe anxiety that is not responsive to conventional treatments. • May cause somnolence, orthostasis. • May contribute to metabolic sx. • Recommended for short-term use only.
Agents to generally avoid	Long-acting benzodiazepines (chlordiazepoxide, diazepam)			• Potential to cause or worsen delirium. • Long half-life may cause significant sedation. • Increased risk for falls.

due to differences in D2 receptor affinity. However, all three of these atypical antipsychotics have the potential to stimulate appetite, cause weight gain, and contribute to the development of the metabolic syndrome. By comparison, aripiprazole and ziprasidone are relatively weight neutral, and may be considered for overweight patients or individuals with comorbidity of hyperglycemia or diabetes. Typical antipsychotics are associated with a higher side effect burden, particularly regarding the risk for EPS and the development of tardive dyskinesia. Clozapine should only be prescribed with the guidance of a psychiatrist with routine monitoring because of the potential for significant side effects, including agranulocytosis.

TABLE 7.5 Antipsychotic Treatments

	Drug or drug class	Starting dose	Maximum dose	Comments
Preferred agents	Risperidone (Risperdal)	0.5 mg daily	2 mg daily (can be given in divided doses)	• Available in dissolvable formulation (M-tab). • Potential for hyperprolactinemia and extrapyramidal symptoms.
	Olanzapine (Zyprexa)	2.5 mg daily	15 mg daily (can be given in divided doses)	• Available in regular PO, dissolvable formulation (Zydis), and IM formulation. • Potential for orthostasis, sedation, weight gain, and other metabolic effects.
	Quetiapine (Seroquel)	25 mg BID	200 mg daily (in divided doses)	• Potential for orthostasis, sedation. • Possibly better tolerated in patients with Parkinson's disease or LBD. • Potential for orthostasis, sedation, weight gain, and other metabolic effects.

TABLE 7.5   (*Continued*)

	Drug or drug class	Starting dose	Maximum dose	Comments
Other agents to consider	Aripiprazole (Abilify)	5 mg daily	20 mg daily	• Available in PO and IM formulations. • Partial dopamine agonist. • Relatively weight neutral.
	Ziprasidone (Geodon)	20 mg BID	60 mg BID	• Available in PO and IM formulations. • Administer with food (500 calories) for enhanced bioavailability. • Relatively weight neutral.
	Haloperidol (Haldol)	1 mg	10 mg daily (in divided doses)	• Available in PO, IM, IV forms. • If administered via IV, telemetry monitoring is required due to risk for Torsades de Pointes.
Agents to generally avoid	Typical antipsychotics Clozapine (Clozaril)			• May have higher risk for developing EPS and TD. • Possibly better tolerated in patients with Parkinson's Disease or LBD. • Should be prescribed under guidance of psychiatrist due to significant side effects (agranulocytosis, risk for seizure, sialorrhea, orthostasis) and mandatory monitoring.

Insomnia

It is not uncommon for hospitalized patients to have difficulty sleeping, for which sedative-hypnotics are prescribed. Geriatric patients can be particularly sensitive to the effects of hypnotic medication. Furthermore, there are certain medications that should be avoided because of the potential to worsen confusion. Table 7.6 lists sleep-inducing treatments. Trazodone, zolpidem, and temazepam are generally utilized for their sedation effects, and carry the least amount of adverse effects among the sedative-hynotic medications. Orthostatic blood pressure should be monitored when trazodone is prescribed. All three agents can increase the risk for falls. Benzodiazepines should be avoided in general because they can worsen the risk for falls and cause confusion. Due to their potential for many side effects, antipsychotics are also avoided. While used in many sleep remedies, anticholinergic medications (e.g., diphenhydramine) can worsen confusion in the elderly.

TABLE 7.6   Sleep-Inducing Treatments

	Drug or drug class	Starting dose	Maximum dose	Comments
Preferred agents	Trazodone (Desyrel)	12.5 mg QHS	150 mg QHS	• Potential for orthostasis, falls.
	Zolpidem (Ambien)	5 mg QHS	10 mg QHS	• Utilize lowest effective dose to minimize risk for falls.
	Temazepam (Restoril)	7.5 mg QHS	30 mg QHS	• Utilize lowest effective dose to minimize risk for falls.
Agents to generally avoid	Benzodiazepines			• Potential for orthostasis, sedation, confusion.
	Antipsychotics (e.g., quetiapine)			• Risks generally outweigh benefit of sedation.
	Anticholinergic medications (e.g., Benadryl)			• Although sedating, it can worsen confusion and risk for side effects outweigh potential benefit.

Behavioral Disturbances Associated with Dementia and Delirium

Dementia and delirium are both associated with a wide variety of behavioral symptoms. One model to conceptualize behaviors proposed by the authors involves clustering the behaviors into one of two broad categories, a hyperactive syndrome and a hypoactive syndrome. These syndromes are not mutually exclusive, and particularly in delirious states, patients may fluctuate between both syndromes.

The hyperactive syndrome is characterized by poor impulse control, behavioral dysregulation and psychomotor restlessness. Examples of this cluster of behaviors include: wandering, yelling, rolling out of bed, and physical aggression. Antidepressants, mood stabilizers, and antipsychotics have all been prescribed to treat "agitation" in patients with dementia. See Table 7.7.

A Black Box Warning has been issued by the FDA for several classes of psychotropic medication used to treat agitation in patients with dementia. One early study providing evidence of increased morbidity in this setting was a meta-analysis examining 17 studies involving atypical antipsychotics [5]. The risk of premature mortality was found to be 1.7 times higher than placebo. Since that time, the elevated risk has been expanded to include typical antipsychotics and valproic acid. The most recent study by Kales et al. noted the relative risk among individual psychotropic medications as follows (listed in descending order for mortality rate with hazard ratio in parentheses): haloperidol (1.59), olanzapine (1.06), risperidone (1.00), valproic acid (0.96), and quetiapine (0.74) [6].

Before initiating intervention for acute agitation, an investigation for the underlying cause must be completed. If immediate action is necessary, the atypical antipsychotics (risperidone, olanzapine, and quetiapine) have been effective for calming the patient. Lorazepam may also be utilized, but note that a paradoxical disinhibition and subsequent worsening of agitation may result. Other alternatives include haloperidol, valproic acid, and trazodone. All of these agents carry the potential to cause side effects.

The hypoactive syndrome is characterized by symptoms of physical inactivity and detachment from surroundings. These patients may present as withdrawn, lethargic, and vacant. They may not respond to or are minimally reactive to environmental stimuli. Severe complications may result, including failure to thrive from inadequate oral intake of food and medications and the formation of decubitus ulcers due to being sedentary. It is common that hypoactive symptoms are not recognized or treated because these patients are less problematic in the hospital setting. It is important to recognize if the cause for the decreased activity is potentially reversible (e.g., depression or delirium).

TABLE 7.7   Acute Agitation Treatments

	Drug or Drug Class	Starting Dose	Maximum Dose	Comments
Preferred agents	Risperidone (Risperdal)	0.25 mg QID prn	2 mg total daily dose	• Available in dissolvable formulation (M-tab). • Potential for hyperprolactinemia and extrapyramidal symptoms.
	Olanzapine (Zyprexa)	2.5 mg QID prn	15 mg total daily dose	• Available in regular PO, dissolvable formulation (Zydis), and IM formulation. • Potential for orthostasis, sedation, weight gain, and other metabolic effects.
	Quetiapine (Seroquel)	12.5 mg QID prn	200 mg total daily dose	• Potential for orthostasis, sedation. • Possibly better tolerated in patients with Parkinson's disease or LBD. • Potential for orthostasis, sedation, weight gain, and other metabolic effects.
	Lorazepam (Ativan)	0.25 mg TID prn	2 mg total daily dose	• Available in PO, IM, and IV formulations. • Drug of choice in patients with liver disease. May cause somnolence, confusion. • Increased risk for falls. • Recommended for short-term use only. • May cause paradoxical agitation/ disinhibition.

TABLE 7.7   (*Continued*)

	Drug or Drug Class	Starting Dose	Maximum Dose	Comments
Other agents to consider	Haloperidol (Haldol)	1 mg	10 mg daily (in divided doses)	• Available in PO, IM, IV forms. • If administered via IV, telemetry monitoring is required due to risk for Torsades de Pointes.
	Valproic acid (Depakote)	125 mg TID prn	1000 mg total daily dose	• Available in regular PO, sprinkles (Depakene), and IV formulations. • Potential for causing sedation, tremor, ataxia. • Monitor for thrombocytopenia, LFT elevations. • Valproic acid levels can be measured. • Potential to raise levels of warfarin.
	Trazodone (Desyrel)	12.5 mg TID prn	150 mg total daily dose	• Potential for orthostasis.

OTHER GERIATRIC CONDITIONS

Parkinson's Disease and Lewy Body Dementia

Parkinson's disease (PD) is a neurological condition involving a deficiency in dopaminergic neurons in the basal ganglia. In addition to the characteristic motor findings of tremor, masked facies, stooped posture, and shuffling gait, psychiatric comorbidity is common. The prevalence of depression among Parkinson's patients is up to 40% [7]. Psychosis is also observed, often exacerbated by the use of dopamine agonists for treatment of the motor symptoms. Lewy body dementia (LBD) patients have similar motor findings of Parkinson's patients along with cognitive impairment and visual hallucinations. Both PD and LBD patients are sensitive to antipsychotic medication.

If the symptoms are severe enough to warrant treatment, the recommended agents are quetiapine and clozapine [8]. Because of the sensitivity to antipsychotics, it is best to start at a low dose and then titrate. Quetiapine can be started at 12.5 mg, and titrated in 12.5 mg increments. If using clozapine, the starting dose should be 6.25 mg given at bedtime. For LBD, there is some evidence that the acetylcholinesterase inhibitor rivastigmine may alleviate some of the psychotic symptoms [9].

CASE STUDY PART 3

After modifying her medications, improving sleep hygiene, and treating potential infections, Mrs. SH remains aggressive and combative, leading to risk of physical harm to herself. Modifications to her physical and social environment have not quieted her behaviors. Consideration may be given to treating with quetiapine, which may be better tolerated in Parkinson's patients for treatment of the psychosis and agitation. Typical antipsychotics should be avoided because it has the potential to worsen parkinsonism. Prior to starting quetiapine, a conversation with the husband or other potential decision-maker should be had explaining the potential risk for premature death associated with antipsychotics and dementia and documented in the chart. The dose of quetiapine should be titrated gradually to clinical effectiveness, while monitoring for oversedation and orthostasis.

Note that delirium may not resolve immediately, even if the underlying cause is discovered and addressed. In other words, there may be a delay in response to the treatment. In the meantime, it may be advisable to assign an attendant to sit with the patient due to her poor insight and judgment, as well as risk for falling due to agitated behavior.

Poststroke Neuropsychiatric Sequelae

Following a stroke, patients are susceptible to personality changes and mood lability, in addition to acute confusion and cognitive changes [10]. In cases of depression, a trial of an antidepressant should be considered (SSRI or SNRI). A more rapid response may result with the use of a psychostimulant [11]. In the event of manic symptoms, valproic acid can be used.

Notably, stroke patients may be predisposed to developing seizures. Partial complex seizures may present as agitated behavior or the patient may even appear psychotic. If the behaviors appear episodic, and a seizure is suspected, an EEG should be obtained. However, it is common that the EEG will not capture epileptiform activity. An elevated prolactin level obtained 30 minutes after the suspected event is also suggestive of a seizure. The appropriate treatment after a seizure is an anticonvulsant.

Pain

Pain becomes more common with increasing age (e.g., osteoarthritis and degenerative disc disease). This can be difficult to assess in the demented patient, who may have difficulty communicating its presence. Moreover, pain may actually be the underlying cause for distress and ultimately leading to disruptive behavior. Specialized scales have been developed to assess pain in this population [12]. In addition, pain medications can contribute to the development or worsening of mental status changes (e.g., meperidine). The SNRIs (duloxetine and venlafaxine) have shown some effectiveness in treating comorbid pain and depression [13]. While TCAs can be used for the same purpose, they are not preferred given the potential for more side effects.

CONCLUSIONS

Evaluation and treatment of behavioral disturbances in the elderly is a complex undertaking. Comprehensive assessment is critical and should include obtaining a thorough history with collateral information to understand baseline functioning, investigating possible reversible causes, and identifying triggers for particular behaviors. In determining whether to utilize a psychotropic medication, the hospitalist must balance the potential benefits with the associated risks. Pharmacological interventions should also be used in combination with behavioral approaches and environmental modifications to address disturbing behaviors. Ongoing monitoring for the emergence of side effects should occur, and a plan developed to taper the medication as soon as possible.

REFERENCES

1. Tune LE. Anticholinergic effects of medication in elderly patients. *J Clin Psychiatry* 2001;62(Suppl. 21):11–14.
2. Inouye SK, Bogardus ST, Charpentier PA, et al. A multicomponent intervention to prevent delirium in hospitalized older patients. *N Engl J Med* 1999;340:669–676.
3. Koenig HG, Meador KG, Cohen HJ, Blazer DG. Depression in elderly hospitalized patients with medical illness. *Arch Intern Med* 1988;148(9):1929–1936.
4. Brink TL, ed. *Clinical Gerontology: A Guide to Assessment and Intervention*. New York: Haworth Press, 1986, p. 113.
5. Schneider LS, Dagerman K, Insel PS. Risk of death with atypical antipsychotic drug treatment for dementia: Meta-analysis of randomized placebo-controlled trails. *JAMA* 2005;294:1934–1943.
6. Kales HC, Kim HM, Zivin K, et al. Risk of mortality among individual antispsychotics in patients with dementia. *Am J Psychiatry* 2012;169:71–79.

7. Starkstein SE, Preziosi TJ, Bolduc PL, Robinson RG. Depression in Parkinson's disease. *J Nerv Ment Dis* 1990;178(1):27–31.

8. Friedman JH, Fernandez HH. Atypical antipsychotics in Parkinson-sensitive populations. *J Geriatr Psychiatry Neurol* 2002;15:156–170.

9. McKeith I, Del Ser T, Spano P, et al. Efficacy of rivastigmine in dementia with Lewy bodies: A randomized, double-blind, placebo-controlled international study. *Lancet* 2000;356(9247):2031–2036.

10. Robinson RG, Starr LB, Kubos KL, Price TR. A two-year longitudinal study of post-stroke mood disorders: Findings during the initial evaluation. *Stroke* 1983;14:736–741.

11. Massand P, Murray GB, Pickett P. Psychostimulants in post-stroke depression. *J Neuropsychiatry Clin Neurosci* 1991;3(1):23–27.

12. Warden V, Hurley AC, Volicer L. Development and psychometric evaluation of the Pain Assessment in Advanced Dementia (PAINAD) scale. *J Am Med Dir Assoc* 2003;4(1):9–15.

13. Lee YC, Chen PP. A review of SSRIs and SNRIs in neuropathic pain. *Expert Opin Pharmacother* 2010;11(17):2813–2825.

CHAPTER *8*

ISSUES AND CONTROVERSIES SURROUNDING NUTRITION IN HOSPITALIZED OLDER ADULTS

Lauren W. Mazzurco
Joseph Murray
Caroline A. Vitale

INTRODUCTION

Eating difficulties, loss of appetite, and poor caloric intake are concerns that develop commonly among hospitalized older adults. These nutritional concerns usually arise in the context of an acute illness, often when the immediate prognosis is unclear. Assessing and managing a frail hospitalized older adult with eating difficulties or poor oral intake is clinically challenging due to the multifactorial nature of these problems. Without clear and immediate remedies, nutritional concerns can often become a vexing clinical challenge, as malnutrition is associated with functional decline and substantial in-hospital morbidity and mortality. Guiding family and caregivers through decision-making with regard to potential benefits, risks, and treatment burdens of alternative forms of nutritional supplementation can also be daunting even to experienced providers. We offer a pragmatic approach to common nutritional concerns that arise among hospitalized older adults that includes careful clinical assessment along with strategies to optimize nutrition and quality of life, while mitigating potential risks and treatment burdens associated with some interventions.

Hospitalists' Guide to the Care of Older Patients, Edited by Brent C. Williams, Preeti N. Malani, and David H. Wesorick.

MALNUTRITION

Malnutrition—also known as protein-calorie malnutrition, protein-energy malnutrition, undernutrition, or marasmus—among older adults is commonplace. While many definitions of malnutrition exist, the following characterization provides an excellent framework relevant for the older hospitalized adult population:

> Protein-energy malnutrition . . . is present when insufficient energy and/ or protein is available to meet metabolic demands . . . and may develop because of poor dietary protein or calorie intake, increased metabolic demands as a result of illness or trauma, or increased nutrient losses. [1]

Those with acute illness, prolonged hospitalization, cognitive impairment, frequent infections, and pressure ulcers are at heightened risk for malnutrition. Estimates indicate that 12–50% of hospitalized older adults are considered to be malnourished [1]. Some are malnourished on admission, and others develop poor oral intake as a result of an acute illness, which, if not addressed, may lead to malnutrition.

NUTRITIONAL ASSESSMENT: GERIATRIC CONSIDERATIONS

Anthropometric measurements take into account changes in body composition and weight that normally occur with aging, including a progressive loss of lean body mass, and replacement with and redistribution of body fat. Often, malnutrition can be identified by simply questioning a patient or their loved ones about recent weight changes. Generally, a loss of more than 5% body weight in 1 month or loss of more than 10% body weight in 6 months are considered significant [2]. Of course, these changes in weight must be addressed in the context of other clinical factors, such as fluid retention and even amputations. Alternatively, Body Mass Index (BMI) may be used for quick assessment; however, this measure must also be interpreted with caution as it can be particularly problematic when assessing older adults, who are more likely to have conditions, such as edema, ascites, kyphoscoliosis, or contractures, that impact height and weight measurements.

Gathering Relevant History

Review of a patient's medical, cognitive, and social history often provides insight into potential causes of malnutrition or poor oral intake. As shown in Table 8.1, information obtained in a routine admission history and

TABLE 8.1   Clinical Approach to Assessment of Poor Oral Intake or Malnutrition in Hospitalized Older Adults

Etiology	Example[a]
Anorexia[b]	
Acute or chronic medical condition	Congestive heart failure
	Chronic obstructive pulmonary disease
	Malignancy
	Infection
	Hyper- or hypothyroidism
	Inflammatory conditions
Dietary restriction or food preferences	Restrictions of sodium, potassium, carbohydrate, protein
	Fluid restriction
	NPO (nothing by mouth) status
	Texture restriction (i.e., pureed, mechanical soft)
Cognitive and/or psychiatric disorders	Dementia
	Delirium
	Depression
	Bereavement
Medications	Polypharmacy
	Adverse effects (xerostomia, dysguesia, nausea)
	Drug-nutrient interactions
Functional impairment	
Physical conditions	Tremor
	Altered dexterity or decreased range of motion
	Neuropathy
	Hemiparesis
	Debility
	Mobility problems/bed bound
	Vision Impairment
Social factors	Social isolation
	Lack of transportation
	Limited or low income
	Substance abuse
	Low literacy
Oropharyngeal/ swallowing problems	Poor dentition or ill-fitting oral appliances
	Stroke
	General weakness/debility
	Dementia
	Xerostomia
	Altered taste sensation
	Oral candidiasis
	Mucositis
	Bradykinesia due to Parkinson's disease

[a]Not meant to be an exhaustive list.
[b]Anorexia—defined here as lack of appetite.

physical exam helps guide healthcare providers to consider etiologies related to one of three general domains associated with poor nutritional intake: anorexia, functional impairment, and oropharyngeal/swallowing problems. For example, a patient may have loss of appetite associated with advanced congestive heart failure and a restricted cardiac diet. Or, altered dexterity related to advancing osteoarthritis in the setting of social isolation can contribute to functional impairment associated with poor nutritional intake. Additionally, many conditions, such as advanced chronic obstructive pulmonary disease or depression, can be associated with both loss of appetite and functional impairment.

Understanding Baseline Functional Status

Exploring a patient's ability to perform activities of daily living (ADLs), such as bathing, grooming, dressing, feeding, and toileting, is essential and offers information about a patient's baseline functional status. Consider a patient with tremor that makes it difficult to prepare food or even feed oneself independently. The patient may not express these difficulties openly, but an appreciation of such physical examination features provides an opportunity to ask the patient about the impact of these changes on daily functioning. Understanding the older adult patient's baseline eating habits prior to hospital admission is also paramount. Knowing whether a patient was independent in eating or dependent on a caregiver for feeding prior to admission will help tailor rehabilitative efforts to encourage oral intake in a hospitalized patient who may be convalescing from an acute illness.

Understanding Baseline Cognitive Status

Understanding the older adult patient's baseline cognitive status prior to hospitalization is equally essential. Often, to gain this information, one must obtain history from family members or caregivers of the patient. These observations can be key to determining whether the patient is currently at baseline with regard to cognitive status, or whether delirium or other etiologies of an altered mental status need to be considered. When a history of dementia is elicited, understanding the stage of dementia will also guide rehabilitative efforts. Functional impairments that result in malnutrition among patients with moderate dementia are often related to difficulties with meal preparation, social isolation, and difficulties with shopping and food procurement. With advanced dementia, the presence of more profound cognitive deficits results in difficulties with using utensils (due to loss of ability to recognize how to use the utensils), and is commonly associated with the development of an oropharyngeal dysphagia or dyspraxia, in which the

TABLE 8.2   Examples of Common Eating Problems among Patients with Dementia

- Losing interest/attention after a few bites
- Holding food in mouth
- Spitting food out
- Batting away spoon presented by feeder
- Perseverative behaviors (e.g., chewing without swallowing)
- Coughing or choking when fed in a semi-recumbent position
- Failing to contain food orally, form a bolus, or move food within the oral cavity
- Experiencing difficulty while chewing or swallowing foods of a particular consistency.

patient is unable to effectively move the food bolus from the oral cavity to the pharynx. Common eating behaviors observed in patients with dementia have been identified [3] and are described briefly in Table 8.2. The diagnosis and assessment of eating behaviors associated with dementia in a hospitalized patient can be particularly challenging, as delirium, either the hypoactive or hyperactive form, is often complicating the clinical picture. Underrecognized and underdiagnosed, delirium is an important contributor to poor nutritional intake during an acute hospitalization (see Chapter 12) as the patient with delirium is unable to volitionally manage eating independently due to inattention and disorientation. When delirium is present, an evaluation aimed at diagnosing and treating contributing and potentially modifiable factors, such as infection, uncontrolled pain, medication adverse effects, hypoxia, and metabolic disturbances, is indicated.

TOOLS USED FOR SCREENING AND AS DIAGNOSTIC AIDS FOR MALNUTRITION

Systematic screening for malnutrition for all hospitalized patients has become standard due to the high prevalence of malnutrition among older adults admitted to the hospital. The Joint Commission for Accreditation of Health Care Organizations (JCAHO) has mandated that hospitals provide nutritional assessment for all patients upon admission that should include screening and subsequent formal evaluation if it is determined that the patient is at increased risk of malnutrition [4, 5]. In most hospital settings, this nutrition screening is accomplished through the nursing admission assessment. Nutritional screening performed upon hospital admission may help to identify not only those patients who are already malnourished, but also those who are at risk of nutritional deficiency during their hospital stay. Information related to anthropometric data, clinical and biochemical evaluation, and review of dietary habits can be helpful in further delineating the degree—and potentially the underlying etiology—of poor oral intake or malnutrition.

Several screening tools have been validated and are available for use in the older hospitalized patient. The Mini-Nutritional Assessment–Short Form (MNA®-SF) [6, 7] is one of the most widely studied and used screening tools and is available in multiple languages (Fig. 8.1). This well-validated, six-question tool may be used as an initial screen. If the score on this six-question screen demonstrates risk for malnutrition, an additional 12 questions are performed to complete the full 18-question Mini-Nutritional Assessment (MNA®) [8–10], to determine if the patient is indeed malnourished. With a reported sensitivity of 96% and a specificity of 98%, the MNA has been shown to be predictive for in-hospital mortality, increased length of stay, and greater likelihood of discharge to a long-term care facility. The MNA correlates with serum albumin levels and number of prescribed medications. This tool has also been shown to be predictive of the risk of malnutrition in those patients who are otherwise healthy even before weight loss occurs. Both steps can be performed quickly as part of the initial nursing assessment or along with the admission history and physical exam. An illustrative case example follows.

CASE STUDY 8.1

Mrs. S. is an 80-year-old retired teacher with a past medical history significant for hypertension, hyperlipidemia, and osteoarthritis. She is now admitted to the hospital for further evaluation and management of chest pain. Widowed 1 year ago, she lives independently, and has supportive grown children who live nearby. She does not drive; however, her children help with her grocery shopping and errands. She was hospitalized 2 months ago for pneumonia; at that time she was started on an antidepressant due to concerns about her depressed mood. Her BMI is 23. As part of the initial nursing assessment, the MNA-SF is performed (see Fig. 8.1). The patient admits to having a moderate loss of appetite during the last 3 months, with decreased food intake, resulting in 1 point being assigned for Part A. She is unsure if there has been weight loss, thus 1 point for Part B. She is able to get out of bed, but rarely goes out, giving her 1 point for Part C. She was hospitalized 2 months ago, which results in 0 points for Part D. There is concern for depression associated with the fairly recent death of her husband, therefore 0 points for Part E. Her BMI is calculated to be 23, which results in 3 points for Part F. Her total score on the MNA-SF based on this information would be 6, which would suggest possible malnutrition. In this case, going on to complete the full MNA would be necessary to determine the malnutrition indicator score, which will aid in establishing whether a patient is at risk for malnutrition or is deemed to have overt malnutrition prompting additional workup.

Mini Nutritional Assessment
MNA®

Nestlé
NutritionInstitute

Last name:			First name:		
Sex:	Age:	Weight, kg:	Height, cm:	Date:	

Complete the screen by filling in the boxes with the appropriate numbers. Total the numbers for the final screening score.

Screening

A   Has food intake declined over the past 3 months due to loss of appetite, digestive problems, chewing or swallowing difficulties?
0 = severe decrease in food intake
1 = moderate decrease in food intake
2 = no decrease in food intake ☐

B   Weight loss during the last 3 months
0 = weight loss greater than 3 kg (6.6 lbs)
1 = does not know
2 = weight loss between 1 and 3 kg (2.2 and 6.6 lbs)
3 = no weight loss ☐

C   Mobility
0 = bed or chair bound
1 = able to get out of bed / chair but does not go out
2 = goes out ☐

D   Has suffered psychological stress or acute disease in the past 3 months?
0 = yes   2 = no ☐

E   Neuropsychological problems
0 = severe dementia or depression
1 = mild dementia
2 = no psychological problems ☐

F1 Body Mass Index (BMI) (weight in kg) / (height in m^2)
0 = BMI less than 19
1 = BMI 19 to less than 21
2 = BMI 21 to less than 23
3 = BMI 23 or greater ☐

IF BMI IS NOT AVAILABLE, REPLACE QUESTION F1 WITH QUESTION F2.
DO NOT ANSWER QUESTION F2 IF QUESTION F1 IS ALREADY COMPLETED.

F2 Calf circumference (CC) in cm
0 = CC less than 31
3 = CC 31 or greater ☐

Screening score (max. 14 points)

12 - 14 points: Normal nutritional status
8 - 11 points: At risk of malnutrition
0 - 7 points: Malnourished ☐☐

References
1. Vellas B, Villars H, Abellan G, et al. Overview of the MNA® - Its History and Challenges. *J Nutr Health Aging*. 2006;**10**:456-465.
2. Rubenstein LZ, Harker JO, Salva A, Guigoz Y, Vellas B. Screening for Undernutrition in Geriatric Practice: Developing the Short-Form Mini Nutritional Assessment (MNA-SF). *J. Geront*. 2001; **56A**: M366-377
3. Guigoz Y. The Mini-Nutritional Assessment (MNA®) Review of the Literature - What does it tell us? *J Nutr Health Aging*. 2006; **10**:466-487.
4. Kaiser MJ, Bauer JM, Ramsch C, et al. Validation of the Mini Nutritional Assessment Short-Form (MNA®-SF): A practical tool for identification of nutritional status. *J Nutr Health Aging*. 2009; **13**:782-788.
® Société des Produits Nestlé, S.A., Vevey, Switzerland, Trademark Owners © Nestlé, 1994, Revision 2009. N67200 12/99 10M
For more information: www.mna-elderly.com

Figure 8.1   The Mini-Nutritional Assessment (MNA®) is a widely used screening tool available in multiple languages. Reprinted with permission from Nestlé Nutrition. Please see http://www.mna-elderly.com for Full MNA.
®Société des Produits Nestlé S.A., Vevey, Switzerland, Trademark Owners.
©Nestlé, 1994, Revision 2009. N67200 12/99 10M.

As illustrated in the case, the MNA is best performed in individuals who are able to provide a reliable self-report, or have loved ones or caregivers who can provide supplemental information. With this in mind, a study comparing three of the most commonly used nutritional screening tools suggests that approximately two thirds of hospitalized older adults can be screened using the MNA, which raises the question of how to screen those who are unable to provide reliable self-report [11]. The Nutritional Risk Screening 2002 (NRS 2002), endorsed for use in hospitalized patients by the European Society for Parenteral and Enteral Nutrition (ESPEN), includes criteria related to factors that affect nutritional status as well as disease severity. Because the NRS 2002 assesses nutritional status by calculation of BMI, percentage of oral intake, or weight loss, it does not require subjective information from the patient and thus may be used in those patients who are unable to provide reliable history. This assessment includes initial screening questions, which, if answered positively, instructs users to complete the final screening questions. This tool, however, does not classify or diagnose malnutrition. Rather, it guides healthcare providers in identifying those patients who may benefit from nutritional supplementation, evaluation, or closer monitoring [12].

FURTHER CLINICAL EVALUATION

Medication Review

Other factors that may negatively affect nutrition need to be considered. Culprits often include new medications. Patients with polypharmacy are at risk for an increased number of adverse effects, including loss of appetite and nausea, as well as effects on swallowing function (e.g., anticholinergic effects associated with xerostomia). Medication review should be part of the evaluation of loss of appetite or malnutrition. Many commonly used medications have been implicated as causes of dysguesia, xerostomia, nausea, or nutritional deficiency. Two common examples include metronidazole, with its associated metallic taste, and steroid inhalers that predispose the patient to oral candidiasis if the oropharynx and dentures are not properly rinsed after use.

At the Bedside: Physical Exam Pearls for Assessing Nutritional Concerns

When examining a hospitalized older adult, information about nutritional status can be gained through brief, yet astute observation. Noting the patient's level of consciousness, position in bed, presence of muscle atrophy and/or contractures, presence of nasal cannula or an oxygen mask, and whether the patient is mouth breathing can provide clues to malnutrition risk. Important information can also be gleaned through a careful examination of the patient's oral cavity. Observing the state of dentition, mucous membranes and oral hygiene is essential, as pain from dental caries, poor oral hygiene and xerostomia can contribute to difficulties with chewing and swallowing.

Clinically, it can be difficult to interpret many physical exam findings when assessing for nutritional deficiency or malnutrition. Subtle changes, such as loss of subcutaneous fat, may be the results of a normal aging process. Thus, clinicians should also consider using more objective information, such as laboratory data. Many of the laboratory studies routinely performed on admission to the hospital may suggest malnutrition or aid in the assessment of nutritional status, as shown in Table 8.3.

Furthermore, specific clinical symptoms and/or certain objective findings suggestive of malnutrition may also warrant additional workup. A useful list of triggers that would support a need for further clinical exploration and search for potential reversible factors contributing to malnutrition are listed in Table 8.4.

DYSPHAGIA, ASPIRATION CONCERNS, AND SWALLOWING EVALUATIONS: PEARLS AND PITFALLS

An important clinical distinction is to attempt to determine if there are concerns about the patient having difficulty swallowing (dysphagia) versus overall poor oral intake or loss of appetite. Clinical signs that can often be observed at the bedside may give clues to the potential presence of dysphagia (Table 8.5). It may also be helpful to obtain the input of a speech-language pathologist to help identify causes for eating difficulties. Unless the patient has reached the advanced stages of dementia, where persistent eating problems occur as part of the terminal stages of this condition, appropriate medical management and feeding/swallowing strategies can help the patient regain baseline function. A speech language pathologist may assist the care team by assessing swallow function in the hospitalized patient. The assessment process can range from a simple bedside screening intended to reveal overt signs of aspiration to a modified-barium swallow or a laryngoscopic evaluation of swallowing. The intent of the assessment should not be limited to identifying aspiration events but rather other underlying conditions that may be targeted for amelioration or compensation in an attempt to make the patient's swallowing safer or more efficient.

TABLE 8.3 Assessing Nutritional Status of Hospitalized Older Adults— Interpreting Common Laboratory Studies

Laboratory study	Comments
Compete blood count Iron Studies	• Anemia • Iron deficiency can result from malabsorption in addition to occult bleeding • Transferrin half-life ~9 days. • Unclear associations with outcomes
Vitamin B12	• Deficiency can be due to poor nutritional intake versus pernicious anemia/malabsorption
Folate	• Deficiency can indicate insufficient dietary intake versus drug effects (e.g., methotrexate)
Complete metabolic panel	• Sodium, calcium, and glucose derangements can be detected
Prealbumin	• Half-life ~2 days • Monitor trend rather than absolute value • Failure to return to normal range from a low level with adequate protein supplementation is a poor prognostic sign
Albumin	• Half-life ~18 days. • Negative acute-phase reactant may be affected by acute illness/infection and therefore difficult to interpret nutritional status based on albumin level alone • Hypoalbuminemia associated with in-hospital mortality, prolonged length of stay, readmissions, and complications[a]
Urinalysis	• Increased specific gravity can be suggestive of dehydration
Thyroid function studies	• May have weight loss due to hyper- or hypothyroidism (increased metabolic demands)
25(OH) vitamin D	• Deficiency associated with falls and debility
Cholesterol	• Decrease of total cholesterol to <120 during admission correlates with increased complications, length of stay, and mortality[a]. • Late marker of malnutrition and may be more useful as a prognostic tool

[a]Omran ML, Salem P. *Clin Geriatr Med* 2002;18:719–736.

Appearance of the Oral Mucosa

The importance of examining the oral cavity of a hospitalized older adult with eating problems cannot be overstated. Oral health is dependent on salivary flow for several essential protective duties. Besides, antimicrobial properties, salivary flow keeps the oral mucosa moist, buffers destructive acids produced by bacteria, washes away plaques, lubricates the food bolus during

TABLE 8.4   Triggers for Additional Evaluation for Malnutrition or Poor Oral Intake

- Weight loss of >5% in 1 month or >10% in 6 months
- Cognitive impairment or recent cognitive decline
- Recent functional decline
- Acute illness or decompensation of chronic medical problem
- Prolonged hospitalization
- Frequent infections
- Pressure ulcers
- Focal oral symptoms (i.e., dysphagia, mucositis, and thrush)
- Substance abuse
- Social isolation
- Dietary restrictions
- Depression

TABLE 8.5   Red Flags Suggesting Possible Dysphagia and Increased Risk of Aspiration

- *Wet gurgly voice quality.* Chronic inability to clear secretions from the laryngeal airway with aspiration of secretions is strongly associated with risk of aspiration pneumonia.
- *Dysarthric speech.* Slow rate of speech with imprecise articulation. Impairment in speech can correlate with dysphagia. Slow or weakened oral structures contribute to poor oral manipulation of foods, resulting in increased work during meals that can result in fatigue before adequate nutrition or hydration is achieved.
- *Weakened volitional or reflexive cough.* A loud volitional cough is usually adequate to clear the airway. Conversely, a quiet cough would indicate a poor ability to clear the airway.
- *Poor dentition.* Poor dentition or missing teeth can compromise mastication and result in the need for a diet with a soft consistency, potentially limiting intake. Poor oral hygiene is associated with painful mastication.
- *Xerostomia.* Dry mouth is often associated with a decrease in taste sensation and inability to lubricate food adequately during mastication.

the oral stage of swallowing, and buffers gastric contents that find their way into the esophagus.

When salivary flow is compromised, oral health is compromised and the risk of systemic disease is elevated. Xerostomia is a condition that is physically unpleasant for patients and can lead to poor oral intake, likely due to a decrease in taste sensation and inability to lubricate food adequately during mastication. Older adults with xerostomia will often perceive the taste and quality of food to be poor. A complaint of dry mouth may seem innocuous enough during the initial clinical evaluation of the patient, but should be a red flag to probe for associated signs of malnutrition.

Xerostomia has effects that go beyond the physical discomfort of a dry mouth and malnutrition. When salivary flow is reduced, particularly from the parotid gland, the pH of the solution is lowered. Lowered pH in the oral cavity allows certain pathogenic organisms to adhere to buccal epithelial cells. The adherence of these pathogens puts the dysphagic patient with aspiration at greater risk of colonization and eventual pneumonia.

Instrumental Assessments

Although instrumental swallowing assessments using fluoroscopic and laryngoscopic technologies are easily accessible to the majority of health-care providers working in acute care settings, these assessments should only be performed on patients who are cognizant and able to follow commands regarding swallowing. Performing instrumental assessments on frail older adults with conditions such as delirium or dementia are not indicated. Provided the patient is alert and can follow directions, either examination can provide an accurate and reliable answer to the simple binary questions regarding the presence or absence of aspiration, penetration of the laryngeal airway by food or liquid, and the presence of retained food after the swallow. Other more complex measures can also be obtained. Although the measurement of movement and the timing of the duration of different events during the process of swallowing have contributed to our understanding of swallow biomechanics, these measures are meager substitutes for swallowing function in clinical practice. Furthermore, the videofluoroscopic swallowing study is time-limited due to radiation exposure. This reduces the opportunity to observe patient performance over an entire meal. Many patients perform well during the first few minutes of feeding but subsequently fatigue and begin to demonstrate signs that would be missed during the short duration of a typical radiological study.

Aspiration Concerns

Aspiration has prevailed as the central focus of the swallowing assessment, perhaps because it can be objectively observed during an imaging study and the often dramatic visualization of this finding. Many clinicians presume that aspiration of food, liquid, secretions, or refluxed gastric contents will induce aspiration pneumonia even though clinical experience may reveal many patients who consistently aspirate yet do not experience repeated episodes of aspiration pneumonia. Still, nothing per oral (NPO) orders continue to be reflexively recommended in anticipation of preventing pneumonia in those patients who aspirate even small amounts. Adequate consideration is often not given to long-term "aspirators" without pneumonia who consistently demonstrate the ability to reflexively clear material from the airway. Some patients who have been safely maintaining nutrition and hydration for years undergo videofluoroscopy or laryngoscopic examinations for the first time, and are ordered to stop eating after aspiration is observed. This not only deprives the patient of the physical pleasure and relief of taking in food and liquid for sustenance, but also commonly results in the placement of an alternate route for nutritional support, such as a feeding tube.

Langmore and coworkers concluded that dysphagia and aspiration are necessary, but not sufficient conditions for the development of aspiration pneumonia [13]. Other factors must be considered, including functional status and health status. These investigators found that patients who were dependent on others for feeding had the greatest odds of acquiring aspiration pneumonia. This makes clinical sense, in that patients who cannot feed themselves are dependent on others—frequently untrained but well-meaning caregivers—who may commence or continue the feeding when the patient is in a state of fatigue, lethargy, inattention, or sedation. Patients dependent for feeding will also likely be dependent for oral care, and a reduction in the frequency or quality of oral hygiene can contribute to the promotion of oral flora that could be harmful if aspirated.

In fact, the control of aspiration through the placement of feeding tubes is closely associated with aspiration pneumonia. It is established that patients with tube feeding will likely continue to aspirate oropharyngeal secretions, and that the oropharyngeal secretions that are produced by patients with tube feeding are more likely to be colonized because direct care staff may not perceive the need to maintain oral hygiene in patients who do not eat orally. Further, aspiration of refluxed tube feedings is not uncommon. Overall, tube feeding carries with it substantial long-term treatment burdens that need to be weighed in the context of the patient's underlying condition, treatment preferences, and potential benefits of having tube feeding [14, 15].

Finally, the quality of life of the patient should not be dismissed. Eating and drinking are fundamental and symbolic biological processes. Being denied this simple and basic drive to satisfy hunger and thirst can be both demeaning and demoralizing. Often, those patients in whom a feeding tube is placed are kept at an "NPO" status indefinitely. In those older adults receiving a feeding tube, proactive reassessment of swallowing abilities and trials of small amounts of food by mouth at later points in time should be encouraged. Further discussion regarding tube feeding decisions in older adults can be found later in this chapter.

Worries about malnutrition are often a primary source of anxiety on the part of patients' caregivers and loved ones, as well as a concern for the medical team caring for the patient. Challenging situations often arise in cases where the patient is not regaining the ability to eat, the overall prognosis is deemed by medical providers to be poor, and continued "full court press" efforts to treat acute medical conditions have come to the point where they are likely no longer helpful, if not futile. In fact, the hospitalist may encounter a situation where it feels as though the treatments being prescribed (e.g., continued broad spectrum IV antimicrobials, daily blood draws, PICC line insertions, daily dressing changes, etc.) are not resulting in improvement in the patient's appetite or functional status, and may no longer be in the patient's best interests. The primary medical team may sense the need to shift the patient's goals of care to those centered on comfort and quality of life, instead of attempts to cure the patient's irreversible medical conditions. These situations often arise when attempting to articulate these points to the patient's family during "goals of care discussions" (see Chapter 5) and efforts to shift to a more palliative approach.

CASE STUDY 8.2

Mrs. M, a 91-year-old woman with moderate to advanced dementia, peripheral vascular disease, osteoarthritis, and osteoporosis, and who has been nonambulatory since a hip fracture six months ago, is admitted to the hospital with sacral pain due to a new pressure ulcer. She had been discharged from a subacute rehabilitation facility approximately 1 month ago to her son's home as her son is her primary caregiver. At baseline, she is dependent on her son for all activities of daily living, including feeding. She is currently being treated with IV antimicrobials for presumed osteomyelitis of the sacrum. She has had minimal oral intake since admission to the hospital 4 days ago despite the nursing staff's attempts to feed her. She has been coughing more frequently, and there is concern that she may have a faint right lower lobe infiltrate on her chest radiograph obtained this morning. Due to concerns about her risk for aspiration, her dietary orders were changed to "NPO." A small-bore nasogastric (NG) tube (e.g., Dobhoff tube) was placed to supplement her nutritional intake. Mrs. M subsequently pulled out the NG tube that evening. Soft wrist restraints were then ordered, and the tube was reinserted. The patient then became agitated and repeatedly cried out in pain. After several trials of adjusting her pain medications, as well as a trial of an antipsychotic medication (haloperidol) for management of agitation related to delirium, further discussions regarding the overall goals of care for Mrs. M were had with the patient's son, who was also the patient's durable power of attorney for healthcare decisions. After several meetings in which the patient's current conditions and overall prognosis was discussed, a shared decision was made to shift the focus of care to center on symptom management and comfort, to optimize Mrs. M's quality of life. Therefore, her NG tube and restraints were removed. Wound care efforts continued and comfort feeding (assisted oral feeding) was pursued as tolerated, without a focus on caloric intake or weight measurements, despite her risk of aspiration. Mrs. M appeared much more comfortable and had no further episodes of agitation during her hospitalization. She was able to take small amounts of pureed food by mouth through careful assisted oral feeding several times per day. She was discharged to a skilled nursing facility to receive ongoing wound care and to finish her IV antimicrobials, with her overall comfort-oriented plan of care in place.

This case illustrates several teaching points worth noting. In essence, the patient's medical team placed the small-bore nasogastric tube to sustain nutrition which in retrospect was likely contributed to this patient's discomfort and agitation. In Mrs. M's case, it can be argued that the placement of the nasogastric tube was a tipping point in her level of discomfort. After witnessing the patient's heightened level of distress, the patient's son was agreeable to removal of the nasogastric tube. Once the tube was removed, the patient became remarkably calm and restraints were removed. She was allowed to resume oral eating with assistance despite a presumed aspiration risk, and the team was able to move forward with an appropriate plan of care for the patient.

For a patient who continues to decline or who has difficulty maintaining oral caloric intake due to altered mental status or delirium, a concern for overt aspiration of food commonly arises. In the short term, this concern is often addressed by the insertion of a temporary small-bore NG tube through the patient's nostril and into the duodenum as a means to allow continued caloric intake often with the intent of avoiding the risk of aspiration of food with swallowing. Although the intent of providers instituting temporary feeding via a small-bore nasogastric tube is usually to "bridge" the patient until the patient can resume eating, this practice can be fraught with difficulties. A nasogastric tube is often placed in an attempt to provide nutrition while avoiding further episodes of overt aspiration, yet the risk of aspiration pneumonia is usually not ameliorated with this intervention, but instead appears to remain higher than without the nasogastric tube [16].

Hospitalists may encounter ethical dilemmas by feeling pressure to provide burdensome care in the face of potentially medically futile situations. Decisions as to whether to place small-bore nasogastric tubes and/or percutaneous endoscopic gastrostomy (PEG) tubes versus supporting continued assisted oral feeding despite the risk of aspiration are among the most challenging and emotionally charged decisions that hospitalists can encounter with patients and families. The current evidence base regarding the utility of feeding tube insertion and subsequent artificial nutrition and hydration among the frail elderly is extrapolated mostly from observational studies of patients with advanced dementia, a terminal condition in which eating problems develop in more than 85% of patients [17]. Although approximately one-third of nursing home patients are fed through a feeding tube, studies have failed to show any benefit with regard to clinically important outcomes, such as functional status, pressure ulcer healing, comfort, or risk of aspiration pneumonia among patients with advanced dementia [18, 19]. One prospective cohort study demonstrated that hospitalized patients with advanced dementia had a high short-term mortality (6-month median mortality 50%) with or without feeding tube placement, and that feeding tube placement had no measurable benefit on survival [20]. It should be noted that these conclusions are drawn from observational data only as there has been no randomized controlled trial of tube feeding versus assisted oral feeding in patients with advanced dementia or other chronic conditions. Nonetheless, these observational data serve as important best evidence, as it would be logistically and ethically difficult to carry out a randomized controlled trial of tube feeding versus assisted oral feeding. For certain conditions, however, such as amyotrophic lateral sclerosis (ALS) and upper gastrointestinal tract anatomic obstruction, there is likely a role for tube feeding to extend life and to contribute to quality of life, as delineated in Table 8.6.

Starvation

When patients have continued poor oral intake, concerns about the potential for eventual starvation often arise not only among family members and patient surrogate decision-makers, but also among healthcare providers. The word "starvation," when applied to patients with terminal illnesses or severe neurological impairment, is emotionally laden, often conjuring up disturbing visual images of listless, gaunt persons, presumably experiencing profound hunger, and from whom food and water are actively being withheld [21]. Worries about starvation and associated discomfort likely factor into decisions to pursue tube feeding in very ill, hospitalized older adults with poor caloric intake. In reality, however, patients with advanced neurological disease or terminal illness (e.g., advanced dementia) are likely to manifest decreased oral intake and rejection of food due to progression of the underlying condition. Teasing out whether there exists a superimposed acute illness or delirium and recognizing the presence of an underlying advanced condition in the midst of an acute hospitalization can be difficult for clinicians who are likely not familiar with the patient at baseline.

MANAGING PERSISTENT EATING PROBLEMS

For patients who have persistent poor oral intake and are dependent on others for feeding, healthcare providers are often faced with having to educate

TABLE 8.6 Benefits and Burdens of Feeding Tube Placement

	Dysphagic stroke (patients with previously good quality of life, high functional status[a] and minimal comorbidities)	Dysphagic stroke (patients with decreased level of consciousness, multiple comorbidities, poor functional status[a] prior to stroke)	Amyotrophic lateral sclerosis (ALS)	Persistent vegetative state (PVS)	General frailty (patients with multiple comorbidities, poor functional status, and failure to thrive)	Advanced dementia (patients needing help with daily care, having trouble communicating, and/or incontinent)	Advanced cancer (Excludes patients with early-stage esophageal and oral cancer)	Advanced organ failure (patients with congestive heart failure renal, or liver failure, emphysema, and anorexia-cachexia syndrome)
Prolongs life	Likely	Likely in the short term Not likely in the long term	Likely	Likely	Not likely	Not likely[b]	Not likely	Not likely
Improves quality of life and/or functional status	Up to 25% regain swallowing capabilities	Not likely	Uncertain	Not likely	Not likely	Not likely	Not likely	Not likely
Enables potentially curative therapy/ reverses the disease process	Not likely	Not likely	Not likely	Not likely	Not likely	Not likely	Not likely	Not likely

Note: This information is based predominately on a consensus expert opinion. It is not exhaustive. There are always patients who prove exceptions to the rule.

Adapted from: Community-Wide Clinical Guidelines on Percutaneous Endoscopic Gastrostomy (PEGs)/Tube Feeding. Rochester Community-Wide Clinical Guidelines Initiative. Monroe County Medical Society, Rochester, New York, December 2007, available at: http://www.compassionandsupport.org/pdfs/patients/advanced/PEGs_FinalGuidelines_12.14.07.pdf.

[a]Functional status refers to activities of daily living. A poor functional status means full or partial dependency in bathing, dressing, toileting, feeding, ambulation, or transfers.

[b]There is a small group of patients who fall into this category whose life could be prolonged.

TABLE 8.7   Benefits and Burdens of Assisted Oral Feeding and Tube Feeding

Potential benefits	Potential burdens
Assisted oral feeding (continued eating)	
• Patient able to continue to enjoy the taste of food	• Feeding a patient by mouth requires more time
• Patient has greater opportunity for social interaction	• Patient/family worry about "not doing everything in their power" to address the feeding problems and/or "starving the patient"
• Patient's wishes and circumstances taken into account in terms of pace, timing, and volume of feeding	• Family/caregivers may feel they are hastening death
Tube feeding	
• Family members/caregivers avoid guilt and conflict associated with choosing other treatment options	• PEG patients may become agitated and often resulting in the use of restraints
• Family members/caregivers given additional time to adjust to possibility of impending death	• Patients with PEG tubes may have the following symptoms, some of which may be caused or exacerbated by tube feeding (diarrhea, vomiting) and some made worse by tube feeding (skin breakdown from diarrhea, pulmonary congestion, aspiration pneumonia)
• Family members/caregivers can maintain hope for future improvement	

family members on the potential benefits and burdens of either comfort feeding (also known as assisted oral feeding, or hand feeding) or administration of artificial nutrition and hydration through tube feeding. Table 8.7 outlines potential benefits and burdens of comfort feeding and tube feeding for older adults. For older adults without decision-making capacity (arguably the majority of acutely ill hospitalized frail elderly), surrogate decision-makers' understanding of these concepts, with careful deliberation of risks, benefits, and long-term treatment burdens are critical for informed decision-making and for facilitating a patient-centered plan of care. In addition to the lack of benefit of feeding tubes on important clinical outcomes for most hospitalized older adults, the risks and burdens of feeding tubes may be particularly problematic among frail patients with multiple advanced chronic conditions who may be near the end of life. Feeding tubes have been associated with increased use of physical restraints, agitation, and the need for pharmacological sedation, all of which can diminish quality of life.

Comfort Feeding

Careful hand feeding (comfort feeding) near the end of life is an alternative to tube feeding for patients with advanced dementia or others deemed to be at risk for aspiration in whom preferences to continue oral intake (despite this risk) have been established [22]. Implicit in comfort feeding is a shift from quantifying caloric intake to a focus solely on the patient's enjoyment of taste for quality of life reasons, in as safe a manner as possible. Comfort feeding involves a nurse, certified nursing assistant, family member, or trained volunteer who feeds patients with cognitive impairment in an individualized and nurturing manner. Feeding continues as tolerated. If the patient or resident shows signs of distress with feeding, attempts at feeding should not be forced. The care plan should call for continued interaction with the patient, including meticulous mouth care, and application of moist mouth swabs for comfort.

Family members and caregivers have an intense need to nurture. Acknowledging the symbolic value of food [23] and helping the patient's family nurture the patient can often be accomplished through comfort feeding where possible. In addition, comfort feeding is a way to assure that measures to reduce aspiration risk are being performed through optimal positioning of the patient while feeding, and attempting feeding when the patient is most alert. The task of hand feeding is time intensive and as a result may place further stressors on caregivers. In addition to engaging the registered dietician and head nurse assigned to the hospital unit, the following should be considered to maximize oral intake:

- Flexible mealtimes to match the patient's moments of hunger and satiety or willingness.
- Allowing self-feeding without the use of utensils (use of "finger foods") where feasible
- Allowing for smaller and more frequent meals rather than fewer larger meals
- Concentrating on the midday meal in patients with dementia, which provides the greatest caloric intake.
- Special training for staff in administering food and fluids
- Adapting staff duties to allow for adequate feeding.

NUTRITIONAL SUPPLEMENTS AND PHARMACOLOGIC AGENTS

Nutritional Supplements

Based on data that link poor nutritional status with worse outcomes in hospitalized older adults, healthcare providers often feel compelled to improve nutritional status using both pharmacologic appetite stimulants (orexigenic agents) and nutritional supplements. There is a paucity of data surrounding use of nutritional supplements and orexigenic agents and even fewer studies that have examined the use of pharmacologic therapies among the frail elderly. Moreover, as discussed earlier, a thoughtful approach to the evaluation of poor oral intake in hospitalized older adults is indicated prior to starting therapy, so that potentially treatable causes may be identified, addressed, and corrected. Reviewing the indications, expected outcomes, and potential side effects of these options is essential to appropriate use of these agents.

A recent meta-analysis [24] and systematic review [25] supports use of protein and energy supplementation for weight gain among those older adult hospitalized patients who are noted to be malnourished at baseline. In this population, it is suggested that use of supplements may decrease overall complications; however, further confirmatory studies are needed. There is no evidence that nutritional supplementation affects other important clinical outcomes, such as quality of life, mood, functional status, or survival. Currently, there is no significant evidence to support the use of nutritional supplementation to improve wound healing.

By collaborating with the hospital dietician, appropriate nutritional supplements can be selected based on the patient's underlying comorbid conditions, as well as caloric needs. Requesting a "diet diary" or daily calorie count quantifies a patient's actual intake rather than using subjective estimates of the portion consumed at mealtime. Once it has been determined that a patient may benefit from the addition of nutritional supplements, the following practical suggestions should be considered. Nutritional supplements should be offered to the patient between meals rather than accompanying a meal so as not to reduce mealtime caloric intake. Hospitalized older adult patients frequently exhibit generalized weakness, may have sensory impairments, including low vision, and often have poor dexterity, making it difficult to drink from the container in which the supplements are packaged. In addition, hospitalized older adults often have difficulty drinking from a straw, often due to decreased muscle strength, coordination, and level of alertness. Delirium, unfamiliar food textures and flavors, as well as acute illness can each contribute to poor oral intake and dependency on others for eating while hospitalized. In these cases, staff should be alerted and provide one-to-one assistance to the patient, offering assisted oral feeding where appropriate. Supplements may be served on ice or, if preferred, mixed with ice cream for enhanced flavor and texture.

Orexigenic Agents

There are few options for adjunctive pharmacologic therapies for appetite stimulation in older adults (Table 8.8). Healthcare providers may often feel

TABLE 8.8 **Commonly Used Pharmacologic Appetite Stimulants**

	Indications	Adverse effects	Recommended initial dosing
Megestrol acetate	FDA approved in HIV- and cancer-related cachexia	VTE, Adrenal Insufficiency if >12 weeks of consistent use	400–800 mg PO daily
Dronabinol	FDA approved in HIV patients. One randomized control trial among patients with dementia [24]	Central nervous system effects (somnolence, hallucinations, confusion)	2.5 mg PO QHS
Mirtazapine	Depression	Sedation, orthostatic hypotension	7.5 mg PO QHS

VTE, venous thromboembolism; PO, by mouth; QHS, at bedtime; QID, four times daily.

pressured by caregivers to address a patient's poor appetite or poor caloric intake. Although providers may reflexively reach for pharmacologic therapies to address these problems, these medications should be used only after thoughtful assessment. Unfortunately, however, medication intervention is often begun without careful consideration of the underlying cause(s) of the patient's poor caloric intake. Clinicians should acknowledge that medications for appetite stimulation in older adults are not FDA approved for use in this manner, and therefore, when prescribed, are used in an off-label manner. Use of these medications is limited by the paucity of studies addressing the use of pharmacotherapeutic agents to address anorexia, cachexia, and weight loss in older adults. A few of the more common pharmacologic agents used in this manner are described.

Megestrol acetate is a synthetic derivative of a naturally occurring progesterone-like agent that has been shown to be efficacious for appetite stimulation and weight gain in cancer- and AIDS-related cachexia. In frail older adults, however, there is limited and inconsistent evidence to support its use. Although more studies are needed, one small randomized placebo-controlled trial among frail nursing home patients with weight loss found no significant differences in weight gain between treatment and control groups at 12 weeks; however, the megestrol-treated patients reported significantly greater improvement in appetite, and well-being [26]. These potential benefits, however, must be balanced carefully in the context of known adverse effects, including increased risk of venous thromboembolism and adrenal insufficiency with prolonged use resulting from corticosteroid-like effects. For these reasons, we do not advocate routine use of megestrol in older adults as a treatment for weight loss or to enhance appetite.

In some individuals, antidepressant medications are associated with side effects of weight gain and appetite stimulation. As many older adults experience depression in addition to poor oral intake and malnutrition, it is common for healthcare providers to sometimes prescribe a low-dose antidepressant such as mirtazapine to treat poor appetite, especially since mirtazapine is generally an effective and well-tolerated antidepressant. Compared with other antidepressants, mirtazapine has been shown to be associated with earlier weight gain (within the first 4 weeks of therapy), though caution must be exercised as orthostatic hypotension can result from antagonistic effects on $\alpha2$ receptors. Currently, there is no evidence to suggest that mirtazapine is efficacious for weight gain in the absence of depression or dementia associated depression [27].

Although dronabinol, a cannabinoid derivative, has demonstrated positive effects on weight gain and appetite, this agent has not been studied in older adults. One study did show weight gain in older adults with Alzheimer's dementia [28]; however, further study is needed before dronabinol can be routinely recommended. Use of dronabinol in older adults has been limited by confusion and delirium commonly experienced by patients during their initial encounter with this medication. Because of its antiemetic effects, dronabinol may play a role in providing benefit in patients who have nausea as an underlying etiology for their poor appetite; however, this medication needs to be used with caution in older adults due to associated adverse effects.

Low-dose growth hormone has been studied as a potential appetite stimulant in otherwise stable older adults; however, based on side effect profile as seen in Table 8.8, growth hormone is not recommended for long-term use or use in frail older adults. Other agents, such as corticosteroids, cyproheptadine, and anabolic agents, among others, are also fraught with side effects and insufficient evidence to support their use [29].

Weighing the relative risks and benefits of each pharmacologic agent can be very challenging in clinical practice. If a patient has undergone a full nutritional assessment and reversible causes have been explored and non-pharmacologic approaches tried (e.g., altering flavors, providing food preferences, implementing assistance with meals, removing anticholinergic medications, etc.), consideration of an orexigenic agent may be reasonable. In patients with depression or in those with dementia with depressive symptomatology, mirtazapine would be the medication of choice. In those without depressive symptoms, megestrol can be considered for short-term (>12 weeks) use; however, side effects, such as increased risk of venous thromboembolism, edema, and adrenal suppression, need to be carefully considered. Until better evidence is available regarding the efficacy and safety of these and newer medications on the horizon, and until we know whether these medications can affect meaningful improvements on patient outcomes such as functional status and quality of life, these medications are not recommended as first-line therapies [29].

Managing Swallowing Difficulties: Compensatory Strategies

Frequently, older patients who demonstrate a delayed swallow may aspirate a rapidly moving thin liquid bolus. Reducing the volume of the thin liquid may allow for the bolus to be safely contained in the oral cavity prior to the onset of the swallow. When food residuals remain in the oropharynx after the initial swallow attempt, the amount of food presented to the patient with each bite/sip should be also be considered. A slight decrease in the amount of food being hand-fed to a patient can result in a relaxed, though prolonged, meal.

The thinner the liquid, the more rapidly it will flow through the pharynx. The key to viscosity adjustment of liquids is to slow the flow of the food bolus just enough so that the pharyngeal stage of the swallow is initiated when the bolus is still in the oral cavity. Although thickened liquids are often ordered when there are concerns about aspiration risk, patients typically do not find nectar and honey- thickened liquids appealing and they often go unconsumed. The potential dehydrating effects of not drinking thickened liquids are real and need to also be considered in hospitalized older adults deemed to be at risk for aspiration. Often, it is helpful to engage the hospital dietician and speech-language pathologist to assist in individualizing and optimizing food consistency and food preferences to enhance intake and minimize risk of aspiration, dehydration, and further nutritional decline.

A chin tuck is a maneuver intended to reduce the likelihood of aspiration due to a latent or delayed swallow (Fig. 8.2). When the chin is tucked toward the chest, the food bolus is contained in the oral cavity for a longer period of time, during which time the pharyngeal stage of the swallow is initiated and the airway protected

CONCLUSION

Nutritional concerns occur commonly in a large majority of hospitalized older adults. Hospitalists and other healthcare providers caring for this population must be well versed in nutritional risk assessment and management of patients with nutritional compromise. Many older adults are admitted with preexisting malnutrition or have comorbid or psychosocial characteristics that place them at increased risk of malnutrition. Furthermore, acutely ill patients often experience nutritional compromise stemming from a myriad of factors, including progressive debility, prolonged periods of minimal caloric intake, and the development of concomitant eating and swallowing

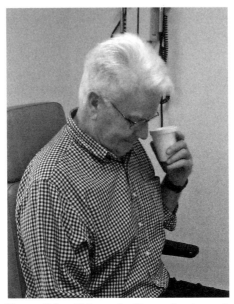

Figure 8.2   Chin tuck. (See color insert.)

problems. In managing patients with eating problems, the skill set of hospitalists must encompass the ability to weigh risks, potential benefits, and treatment burdens when considering various feeding strategies, to elicit patient preferences, and to participate in shared decision-making with older adults or their surrogate decision-makers. Hospitalists are important frontline providers whose practices with regard to nutritional assessment and management can profoundly impact patient outcomes, including quality of life of older adults long after hospitalization.

REFERENCES

1. Wallace JI. Chapter 40: Malnutrition and enteral/parenteral alimentation. In: Halter JB, Ouslander JG, Tinetti ME, Studenski S, High KP, Asthana S (eds.), *Hazzard's Geriatric Medicine and Gerontology*, 6th ed. New York: McGraw-Hill, 2009, pp. 469–481.
2. Ham RJ Indicators of poor nutritional status in older Americans. Report of nutrition screening 1: towards a common view. A consensus conference sponsored by the Nutrition Screening initiative. Washington, DC: Nutrition Screening Initiative; 1991.
3. Blandford G, Watkins LB, Mulvihill MN. Assessing abnormal feeding behavior in dementia: A taxonomy and initial findings. In: Vellas B, Riviere S (eds.), *Weight Loss and Eating Behavior Disorders in Alzheimer's Disease*. New York: Springer, 1998, pp. 47–64.

4. JCAHO Board of Directors. *1995 Comprehensive Accreditation. Manual for Hospitals.* Oakbrook, IL: JCAHO, 1994.

5. Kudsk KA, Reddy SK, Sacks GS, Lai HC. Joint Commission for Accreditation of Health Care Organizations guidelines: Too late to intervene for nutritionally at-risk surgical patients. *JPEN J Parenter Enteral Nutr* 2003;27:288–290.

6. Rubenstein LZ, Harker JO, Salvà A, Guigoz Y, Vellas B. Screening for undernutrition in geriatric practice: Developing the short-form mini-nutritional assessment (MNA®-SF). *J Gerontol A Biol Sci Med Sci* 2001;56:M366–M372.

7. Kaiser MJ, Bauer JM, Ramsch C, et al. Validation of the Mini Nutritional Assessment Short-Form (MNA®-SF): A practical tool for identification of nutritional status. *J Nutr Health Aging* 2009;13:782–788.

8. Van Nes MC, Herrman FR, Gold G, Michesl JP, Rizzoli R. Does the Mini Nutritional Assessment predict hospitalization outcomes in older people? *Age Ageing* 2001;30:221–226.

9. Vellas B, Villars H, Abellan G, et al. Overview of the MNA®—Its history and challenges. *J Nutr Health Aging* 2006;10:456–465.

10. Guigoz Y. The mini-nutritional assessment (MNA®) review of the literature—What does it tell us? *J Nutr Health Aging* 2006;10:466–487.

11. Bauer JM, Vogl T, Wicklein S, et al. Comparison of the Mini Nutritional Assessment, Subjective Global Assessment, and Nutritional Risk Screening (NRS 2002) for nutritional screening and assessment in geriatric hospitalized patients. *Z Gerontol Geriatr* 2005;38:322–327.

12. Kondrup J, Allison SP, Elia M, Vellas B, Plauth M. ESPEN Guidelines for Nutrition Screening 2002. *Clin Nutr* 2003;22:415–421.

13. Langmore SE, Terpenning MS, Schork A. Predictors of aspiration pneumonia: How important is dysphagia? *Dysphagia* 1998;13:69–81.

14. Teno JM, Mitchell SL, Kuo SK, et al. Decision-making andoutcomes of feeding tube insertion: A five-state study. *J Am Geriatr Soc* 2011;59:881–886.

15. Teno JM, Gozalo P, Mitchell SL, Kuo S, Fulton AT, Mor V. Feeding tubes and the prevention or healing of pressure ulcers. *Arch Intern Med* 2012;172:697–701.

16. Finucane TE, Bynum JPW. Use of tube feeding to prevent aspiration pneumonia. *Lancet* 1996;348:1421–1424.

17. Mitchell SL, Teno JM, Kiely DK, et al. The clinical course of advanced dementia. *N Engl J Med* 2009;361:1529–1538.

18. Callahan CM, Haag KM, Weinberger M, et al. Outcomes of percutaneous endoscopic gastrostomy among older adults in a community setting. *J Am Geriatr Soc* 2000;48:1048–1054.

19. Finucane TE, Christmas C, Travis K. Tube feeding in patients with advanced dementia: A review of the evidence. *JAMA* 1999;282:1365–1370.

20. Meier DE, Ahronheim JC, Morris J, Baskin-Lyons S, Morrison RS. High short-term mortality in hospitalized patients with advanced dementia: Lack of benefit of tube feeding. *Arch Intern Med* 2001;161:594–599.

21. Ahronheim JC, Gasner MR. The sloganism of starvation. *Lancet* 1990;335:278–279.

22. Palecek EJ, Teno JM, Casarett DJ, et al. Comfort feeding only: A proposal to bring clarity to decision-making regarding difficulty with eating for persons with advanced dementia. *J Am Geriatr Soc* 2010;58:580–584.

23. Gillick MR, Volandes AE. The standard of caring: Why do we still use feeding tubes in patients with advanced dementia? *J Am Med Dir Assoc* 2008;9:364–367.

24. Milne AC, Avenell A, Potter J. Meta-analysis: Protein and energy supplementation in older people. *Ann Intern Med* 2006;144:37–48.

25. Milne AC, Potter J, Vivanti A, Avenell A. Protein and energy supplementation in elderly people at risk for malnutrition. *Cochrane Database Syst Rev* 2009, CD003288.

26. Yeh SS, Lovitt S, Schuster MW. Usage of megestrol acetate in the treatment of anorexia-cachexia syndrome in the elderly. *J Nutr Health Aging* 2009;13:448–454.

27. Fox CB, Treadway AK, Blaszczyk AT, Sleeper RT. Megestrol acetate and mirtazapine for the treatment of unplanned weight loss in the elderly. *Pharmacotherapy* 2009;29: 383–397.

28. Volicer L, Stelly M, Morris J, McLaughlin J, Volicer BJ. Effects of dronabinol on anorexia and disturbed behavior in patients with Alzheimer's disease. *Int J Geriatr Psychiatry* 1997;12:913–919.

29. Yeh SS, Lovitt S, Schuster M. Pharmacological treatment of geriatric cachexia: Evidence and safety in perspective. *J Am Med Dir Assoc* 2007;8:363–377.

CHAPTER 9

HIP FRACTURE: MANAGING THE MEDICALLY COMPLEX, OLDER SURGICAL PATIENT

Paul J. Grant

INTRODUCTION

Hip fracture patients experience high rates of morbidity and mortality among the geriatric population. Furthermore, many hip fracture patients have multiple chronic medical comorbidities. These facts have elicited hospitalists to become increasingly involved in the care of such patients during the acute hospitalization. The role of the hospitalist spans the entire hospital stay, including the preoperative assessment, instituting perioperative risk reduction strategies, and diagnosing and managing postoperative complications should they arise. The hospitalist also helps ensure a timely and safe transition of care from the inpatient to the outpatient setting. This entire process requires effective communication with the multidisciplinary team, including orthopedic surgery, nursing, and physical and occupational therapy. Box 9.1 summarizes some of the key hospitalist interventions in the care of a hip fracture patient.

EPIDEMIOLOGY

The term "hip fracture" generally refers to any fracture of the proximal femur. Specific classifications include fractures of the femoral neck, intertrochanteric region, and subtrochanteric region (Fig. 9.1). Femoral neck and intertrochanteric fractures are roughly equal in incidence and account for approximately 90% of all hip fractures [1]. These fractures can be classified as "low-energy" fractures that occur with an event such as falling from a

Hospitalists' Guide to the Care of Older Patients, Edited by Brent C. Williams, Preeti N. Malani, and David H. Wesorick.
© 2013 by John Wiley & Sons, Inc. Published 2013 by John Wiley & Sons, Inc.

BOX 9.1

A CHECKLIST OF KEY HOSPITALIST INTERVENTIONS FOR HIP FRACTURE PATIENTS

Preoperative care
- Prescribe pharmacological VTE prophylaxis for most patients who will not proceed immediately to surgery (see Table 9.2).
- Complete a thorough evaluation of the patient, including an assessment of comorbidities. Avoid screening for occult disease (i.e., coronary artery disease), but do optimize medical therapy, when appropriate. Expedite surgery within 24–48 hours, if possible, but recognize that longer surgical delays may be appropriate if required to manage specific clinical conditions.

Postoperative care
- Prescribe pharmacological venous thromboembolism prophylaxis for most patients (see Table 9.2). Continue this for up to 35 days postoperatively.
- Employ delirium prevention strategies, and recognize delirium promptly when it occurs (see also Chapter 12).
- Remove the urinary catheter on postoperative day 1 or 2.
- Manage pain aggressively, but with awareness of the complications of opioid medications, including delirium and constipation.
- Recognize postoperative blood loss anemia, but reserve red blood cell transfusion for symptomatic patients, or those with hemoglobin levels <8 g/dL.
- Involve a physical therapist early in the postoperative care of the patient to hasten mobilization and to assist with discharge planning.
- Assure that all hip fracture patients are discharged on appropriate calcium and vitamin D supplementation.

standing position [2]. Subtrochanteric fractures account for the remaining 10% of hip fractures, and typically arise from higher-energy trauma.

Hip fractures account for an estimated 350,000 hospital admissions annually in the United States. The estimated 30-day mortality associated with hip fractures is 5.2% for women and 9.3% for men. At 1 year, mortality jumps to a staggering 21.9% for women and 32.5% for men [3]. Although hip fracture associated mortality in patients aged 65 and older may be declining, the number of comorbidities in this patient population has increased [3]. Additionally, up to 25% of adults who lived independently prior to their hip fracture require some type of nursing home stay for minimum of 1 year after their injury [4]. Despite recognizing that hip fractures pose a high mortality risk, our ability to objectively predict individual risk is limited. However, a

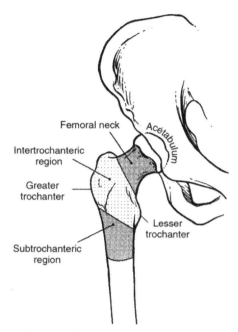

Figure 9.1   Location of various fractures about the proximal femur (or "hip" fractures).

TABLE 9.1   Risk Factors for Hip Fracture

Female gender	Osteoporosis
Advanced age	Low body mass index (BMI)
Caucasian race	Physical inactivity
Malnutrition	Glucocorticoid therapy
Excessive alcohol and caffeine intake	Dementia
Current cigarette smoking	Personal history of hip fracture

recent retrospective analysis of hip fracture patients found that a Charlson Comorbidity Index (an index consisting of 19 major medical comorbidities) of ≥6, age >90 years, and body mass index (BMI) <18.5 correlated with a significantly higher incidence of 30-day postoperative mortality [5].

Major risk factors for hip fracture include advanced age, Caucasian race, osteoporosis, malnutrition, and female gender, with women having a threefold higher incidence than men. These and other risk factors for hip fractures are listed in Table 9.1. Another potential risk factor for osteoporosis-related fractures, including hip fractures, is long-term exposure to the commonly prescribed proton pump inhibitors (PPI). A retrospective trial using a large administrative database demonstrated that PPI exposure for ≥5 years was associated with increased hip fracture risk [6]. A more recent meta-analysis of observational studies found a modest association between PPI use and increased hip and vertebral fractures, but did not find a duration effect of PPI exposure in subgroup analysis [7]. Further studies will be needed to determine if PPIs are truly a risk for osteoporosis-related hip fractures.

With the exception of employing strategies to prevent and treat osteoporosis, methods of preventing hip fractures are extremely limited. Hip protectors are one of the only interventions that have been studied but their efficacy has not been clearly established. A 2010 Cochrane review on the use of hip protectors for preventing hip fractures in older people found a marginally significant hip fracture risk reduction [8]. However, statistical significance was lost after excluding studies considered to be at high-risk of bias. Furthermore, long-term adherence of using hip protectors was noted to be poor.

MODELS OF CARE: THE ROLE OF THE HOSPITALIST

The hospitalist may have various roles when involved with the care of an orthopedic surgery patient. The primary models of care for hospitalists are as follows:

- Attending of record
- Comanager with orthopedic surgery attending
- Traditional consultant.

In one of the first trials to assess the comanagement model of care for hip fracture patients, Phy et al. demonstrated that patients admitted to an orthopedic surgery/hospitalist comanagement service experienced decreased time from admission to surgery, as well as a shortened length of hospital stay, but no differences in inpatient deaths or 30-day readmission rates were observed [9]. In a follow-up study, this group reported that despite improved efficiency and reduced length of stay, patients in the hospitalist comanagement group had no difference in long-term mortality [10].

A retrospective study comparing the use of a hospitalist consult service to a traditional consult service using a primary care physician for hip fracture patients demonstrated a significant reduction in time to consultation and time to surgery with hospitalist involvement [11]. Additionally, there was a trend toward decreased length of stay and total hospital cost in the hospitalist consult group, but this was not statistically significant. More recently, a retrospective cohort study compared hip fracture patients being comanaged daily by a geriatrician and orthopedic surgeon to a "usual care" model of staffing [12]. After adjusting for baseline characteristics, patients in the comanaged group had significantly shorter times to surgery, shorter length of stay, fewer cardiac complications, and fewer cases of infection, delirium, and thromboembolism. No differences were seen in inpatient mortality or 30-day readmission rates.

In summary, hospitalists can have varied roles in the care for hip fracture patients. Although there are few studies that have evaluated how hospitalists affect the outcomes of hip fracture patients, the data currently suggest that hospitalist involvement may improve specific outcome measures. Irrespective of the model of care employed, it is important that the multidisciplinary team (i.e., hospitalist, orthopedic surgeon, geriatrician, nurse, and physical/occupational therapist) work together and communicate effectively to provide optimal care for hip fracture patients.

PREPARING FOR HIP FRACTURE SURGERY

Surgical Options and Optimal Timing for Surgical Repair

The primary goal of hip fracture treatment is to have the patient return to his or her prefracture baseline level of function. This is normally achieved with surgical intervention followed by early mobilization. However, before one can proceed with surgical repair, several factors need to be taken into consideration, including the type of hip fracture, the medical stability of the patient, and the availability of operative time.

The timing of surgery and the surgical repair technique depends on many characteristics of the fracture including the location, whether there is displacement or comminution, and bone quality. A nondisplaced or impacted femoral neck fracture can be repaired by internal fixation or percutaneous pinning (Fig. 9.2). These fractures are preferably repaired within 6 hours as further delay can lead to displacement, which increases the risk for nonunion followed by avascular necrosis of the femoral head [2]. If patients with an impacted femoral neck fracture do not present within 12–24 hours, or present with a fracture that is unstable for more than 24 hours after the injury, a total hip arthroplasty is typically recommended (i.e., replacement of both the femoral head and the acetabulum; Fig. 9.3). Displaced femoral neck fractures, on the other hand, require either a hemiarthroplasty (i.e., prosthetic replacement of the femoral head; Fig. 9.4) or a total hip arthroplasty given the risk of avascular necrosis.

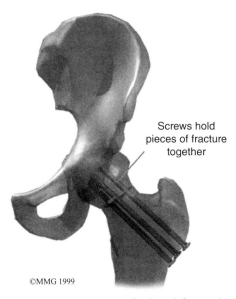

Figure 9.2   Percutaneous pinning of a nondisplaced femoral neck fracture. Image courtesy of Medical Multimedia Group LLC, www.eOrthopod.com.

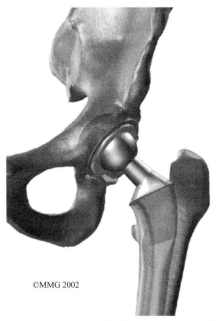

Figure 9.3   Total hip arthroplasty (prosthetic replacement of femoral head and acetabular lining). Image courtesy of Medical Multimedia Group LLC, www.eOrthopod.com.

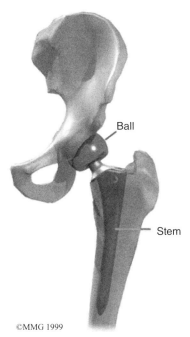

Ball

Stem

©MMG 1999

Figure 9.4   Hemiarthroplasty (prosthetic replacement of the femoral head). Image courtesy of Medical Multimedia Group LLC, www.eOrthopod.com.

Intertrochanteric and subtrochanteric hip fractures pose less risk for osteonecrosis of the femoral head, as these areas of the proximal femur are well vascularized. Intertrochanteric hip fractures, when minimally displaced, can be treated with a variety of internal fixation options, including a sliding hip screw (Fig. 9.5). Surgical repair for subtrochanteric hip fractures, however, typically requires a more extensive procedure such as a total hip arthroplasty (Fig. 9.3) [1, 2].

The optimal timing for hip fracture surgical repair remains somewhat controversial as clinical trials addressing this issue have been inconclusive. Given there are no published randomized controlled trials evaluating the association between timing of hip fracture surgery and mortality, one must rely on observational studies to provide the best evidence currently available.

In a large retrospective study of 8383 consecutive hip fracture patients who underwent surgical repair, there was no difference in adjusted short-term or long-term mortality in patients who underwent surgery 24–48 hours after hospital admission when compared with those undergoing surgery more than 96 hours after admission [13]. There was, however, a lower incidence of pressure ulcers when surgery was performed within 72 hours. A prospective

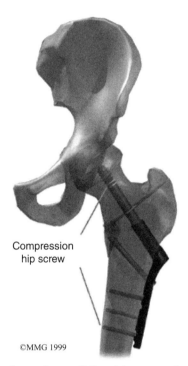

Compression
hip screw

©MMG 1999

Figure 9.5 Internal fixation using a sliding hip screw for an intertrochanteric hip fracture. Image courtesy of Medical Multimedia Group LLC, www.eOrthopod.com.

cohort study of 1178 patients admitted for hip fracture found earlier surgery (defined as <24 hours) was not associated with improved mortality or post-operative function [14]. However, the authors did demonstrate an association between early surgery and significant reductions in pain and hospital length of stay. Similarly, a prospective study by Al-Ani et al. showed no mortality benefit, but did report that early surgical repair was associated with a reduced risk of pressure ulcers and a greater likelihood of returning to independent living after adjusting for several possible confounders [15].

Conversely, multiple observational studies have reported reduced mortality rates in patients undergoing early surgical repair for hip fracture. A retrospective review with multivariate analysis of 651 consecutive hip fracture patients revealed a 1.6-fold increase in 1-year mortality for patients with a surgical delay beyond 48 hours [16]. A review of 129,522 hospital admissions for femoral neck fractures in England reported that a surgical delay of more than 24 hours was associated with an increased risk of in-hospital death [17]. Morrison et al. reviewed 11 studies of mostly medically stable patients and concluded that surgical repair of hip fractures within 24–48 hours of admission is associated with a decrease in 1-year mortality [18]. The investigators also noted that the data are difficult to interpret because most of the studies did not control for the presence and severity of medical comorbidities.

Shiga et al. performed a meta-analysis that included 16 trials and 257,367 patients [19]. These authors found a 41% increased odds of 30-day mortality and a 32% increased odds of 1-year mortality when surgery was delayed for more than 48 hours from time of hospital admission. Another systematic review and meta-analysis identified 16 observational studies involving 13,478 hip fracture patients and concluded that irrespective of the cutoff used to define surgical "delay" (24, 48, or 72 hours), early surgery was associated with a significant decrease in mortality [20]. Furthermore, unadjusted data demonstrated that in-hospital pneumonia and pressure sores were also significantly reduced with early surgery.

A recent prospective cohort study of 2250 consecutive hip fracture patients also determined that delayed surgery carries a higher mortality risk, but found this is largely due to a patient's underlying medical condition causing the delay, rather than the delay itself [21]. Among patients with surgical delay beyond 48 hours, one-third of cases were due to acute medical problems with the need to interrupt antiplatelet therapy accounting for half of these cases. The authors also noted that very long delays in surgery (>120 hours) were associated with worse adjusted outcomes regardless of the reason for the delay.

In summary, the medical literature suggests that surgical repair of hip fractures within 48 hours may improve clinical outcomes in medically stable patients. This may include a decreased risk of mortality (short-term and long-term), shorter length of hospital stay, a reduced risk of pressure ulcers, and an increased likelihood of returning to independent living. It is important to note that surgical delay may be necessary if medical optimization is clinically required. Given that the elderly hip fracture population is often medically complex, delaying surgery to optimize important medical issues is appropriate before proceeding with surgery.

The Preoperative Medical Evaluation for Patients Undergoing Hip Fracture Repair

Regardless of the role in the care of a hip fracture patient (attending of record, comanager, or traditional consultant), hospitalists are well suited to provide an effective and timely preoperative assessment. It is not uncommon for this patient population to have multiple medical comorbidities, such as coronary artery disease, diabetes, hypertension, and chronic kidney disease. Moreover, the circumstances surrounding the hip fracture may require evaluation (i.e., syncope from a cardiac or neurological etiology). Additionally, hip fracture patients are occasionally found "down" for an unknown period of time. This increases the risk for rhabdomyolysis, dehydration, acute renal failure, malnutrition, and electrolyte disturbances. In these cases, medical optimization is required to minimize the risk of perioperative complications.

Hip fracture surgery should be classified as "urgent" surgery. This is surgery that is neither emergent nor elective, but is typically performed during the current hospitalization. As previously stated, hip fracture repair should be performed within 24–48 hours of hospital admission; however, a longer delay may be indicated depending on the patient's clinical presentation. For hip fracture cases, the goal of the preoperative assessment is to identify any unstable cardiac or pulmonary conditions that may influence management. However, there is no role for testing to identify occult disease even when patients have significant risk factors. There are no data to support extensive testing or interventions for clinically stable patients in this setting [22].

For patients who are deemed clinically stable, it is still important to carry out a formal preoperative cardiovascular risk assessment using an objective tool, such as the Revised Cardiac Risk Index (RCRI) [23]. The RCRI is a modern, simple, and prospectively validated system that was developed after studying 4315 patients undergoing major noncardiac surgery. These criteria are virtually identical to the risk factors used in the American College of Cardiology/American Heart Association (ACC/AHA) guidelines on perioperative cardiovascular evaluation for noncardiac surgery [24]. The RCRI include six independent predictors of perioperative cardiovascular complications, which are as follows:

- Ischemic heart disease
- Congestive heart failure
- Cerebrovascular disease (stroke or transient ischemic attack)
- Diabetes mellitus requiring insulin therapy
- Serum creatinine ≥2 mg/dL
- High-risk surgery defined as intraperitoneal, intrathoracic, or suprainguinal vascular surgery (note that a patient undergoing hip fracture surgery will not receive a point for this criteria).

By simply summing these criteria, patients are stratified into low (0–1 risk factor), intermediate (2 risk factors), or high risk (≥3 risk factors) for perioperative cardiovascular complications.

Given the poor positive predictive value of noninvasive stress testing on perioperative cardiovascular events [24], as well as the absence of data demonstrating any benefit of preoperative revascularization [25, 26], the preferred approach to perioperative risk reduction is to medically optimize patents and consider initiating pharmacological therapies when indicated. In high-risk patients, starting beta-blocker therapy one or more days prior to surgery is a recommended approach to decrease perioperative cardiovascular risk. Initiating moderate dose statins prior to surgery is also a reasonable intervention for patients who have an existing indication for this class of medication.

Given that extensive preoperative cardiovascular testing is not recommended, and taking into account that opting not to perform surgical repair of a hip fracture will essentially result in a permanently nonambulatory patient, one could question the utility of performing a preoperative cardiovascular assessment. Even though the vast majority of hip fracture patients will appropriately opt for surgical intervention, it should be noted that risk stratification allows for the patient, the patient's family, and all members of the healthcare team (surgeon, anesthesiologist, etc.) to be informed of the operative risk. For very high-risk patients, the orthopedic surgeon may choose to perform a less invasive procedure, such as percutaneous pinning. Alternatively, if the surgical risk is unacceptably high, or if the patient is already severely limited or bed bound, it may be reasonable to forgo surgery altogether and focus solely on pain control and joint stability, which allows for a patient to be transferred or turned while in bed.

Although an extensive preoperative cardiovascular evaluation is generally not recommended prior to hip fracture surgery, optimization of any active medical issues is appropriate. This may include the medical management of electrolyte disturbances, hydration status, hemodynamic irregularities, hematological abnormalities/coagulopathies, and optimization of any preexisting medical conditions (i.e., chronic obstructive pulmonary disease or congestive heart failure). Limited retrospective data have shown that medical optimization prior to hip fracture surgery is beneficial and does not increase risk from surgical delay.

In summary, there is little role for extensive preoperative evaluation before hip fracture surgery. Hospitalists should evaluate for active, yet treatable, medical issues. If there are no active medical issues, an evaluation for occult cardiac disease is not warranted. In almost all cases, the benefits of hip fracture surgery outweigh the potential risks.

POSTOPERATIVE CARE

Venous Thromboembolism Prophylaxis for Hip Fracture Patients

Among all hospitalized patients, hip fracture patients are among the highest risk for developing venous thromboembolism (VTE). This is due to the multiple risk factors this patient population carries, including advanced age, surgery, trauma, immobility, and the possibility of having comorbid conditions that increase VTE risk, such as congestive heart failure or cancer. Without prophylaxis, the incidence of deep vein thrombosis (DVT) diagnosed by venography in hip fracture patients ranges from 46% to 75% in prospective randomized controlled trials [27–30]. A prospective audit of 580 consecutive hip fracture patients in Britain reported a fatal pulmonary embolism (PE) rate of 4% in patients not receiving prophylaxis versus no fatal PEs among patients receiving thromboprophylaxis [31]. Given these numbers, it is clear that all hip fracture patients require some form of VTE prophylaxis.

Mechanical VTE prophylaxis options include intermittent pneumatic compression (IPC) devices, graded compression stockings, and venous foot pumps. Although the data for mechanical prophylaxis methods in hip fracture patients are very limited, they serve a role in cases where exposure to anticoagulation is contraindicated, or can be used in conjunction with pharmacological prophylaxis. A prospective randomized trial in Canada evaluated IPC devices among 231 trauma patients who suffered a hip fracture [32]. The DVT rate was 4% in the IPC group versus 12% among controls, a statistically significant difference. The 2012 American College of Chest Physicians (ACCP) Guidelines for Prevention of VTE in Orthopedic Surgery Patients [33] only recommends using IPC devices in combination with drug prophylaxis during the hospital stay, or as monotherapy for patients at an increased risk for bleeding.

The ACCP Guidelines for Prevention of VTE gives a strong recommendation for low molecular-weight heparin (LMWH), low-dose unfractionated heparin (LDUH), fondaparinux, warfarin (INR goal, 2–3), and aspirin for VTE prophylaxis in hip fracture patients [33]. Although many factors may influence the choice of thromboprophylaxis, these guidelines favor the use of LMWH (i.e., enoxaparin or dalteparin) over the other agents (see Table 9.2). The newer oral anticoagulant, rivaroxaban (a factor Xa inhibitor), was approved by the U.S. Food and Drug Administration for the prevention of VTE following hip or knee replacement surgery. Rivaroxaban does not currently, however, have an indication for VTE prophylaxis for hip fracture patients. Other new oral anticoagulants, including apixaban (also a factor Xa inhibitor) and dabigatran (a direct thrombin inhibitor), have not been approved for VTE prophylaxis in orthopedic surgery patients in the United States at the time of this writing.

Hip fracture patients are a unique population when it comes to the initiation and duration of pharmacological VTE prophylaxis. Because many hip fracture patients do not undergo surgery for 24–48 hours or more after hospital arrival, initiation of VTE prophylaxis must occur at the time of hospital admission. Furthermore, there is often a delay in presentation to the

TABLE 9.2   VTE Prophylaxis Strategies for Hip Fracture Patients

Drug	Recommended dosing	ACCP level of evidence[a]	FDA approval
LMWH			
Enoxaparin	40 mg sq daily	1B[b]	No
Dalteparin	5000 units sq daily	1B[b]	No
	With either agent:		
	• Not to be given within 12 hours before surgery		
	• First postoperative dose to be given at least 12 hours after surgery.		
LDUH	5000 units sq three times daily	1B	No
Fondaparinux	2.5 mg sq daily	1B	Yes
Warfarin	Dosed to an INR goal of 2–3	1B	Yes
Aspirin	Dose not specified[c]	1B	No
IPC device	Portable, battery-powered devices are recommended to be worn at least 18 hours daily	1C	Manufacturer-specific
	• For use with patients at high risk for bleeding	2C 2C	
	• For use in combination with antithrombotic agent		

Data from: Falck-Ytter et al. [33].
[a]Level of evidence scale: 1 = strong recommendation, 2 = weak recommendation, A = high quality evidence, B = moderate quality evidence, C = low or very low quality evidence.
[b]ACCP recommends use of LMWH in preference over the other drug options listed.
[c]American Academy of Orthopedic Surgeons guidelines recommends an aspirin dose of 325 mg twice daily. A commonly cited large, randomized controlled trial of aspirin versus placebo in hip fracture patients used a dose of 160 mg daily [34].
ACCP, American College of Chest Physicians; FDA, U.S. Food and Drug Administration; INR, international normalized ratio; LMWH, low-molecular weight heparin; LDUH, low-dose unfractionated heparin; IPC, intermittent pneumatic compression; VTE, venous thromboembolism; sq, subcutaneously.

hospital after the injury has occurred. This leaves these high-risk patients, who are typically elderly and now immobile, unprotected from VTE. A prospective study of 133 hip fracture patients revealed a venographically diagnosed preoperative DVT rate of 55% in patients who presented to the hospital more than 48 hours after hip fracture versus 6% in those presenting sooner than 48 hours ($P < 0.001$) [35]. Another trial of 61 consecutive hip fracture patients reported a preoperative DVT rate of 62% in those whose surgery was delayed for 48 hours or more [36]. As such, the risk for VTE in hip fracture patients starts at the time of injury rather than the time of surgery.

The duration of VTE prophylaxis for hip fracture patients was best addressed in a multicenter, randomized, double-blind study of 656 patients [37]. In this study, all patients received once-daily subcutaneous fondaparinux 2.5 mg for 6–8 days postoperatively followed by randomization to either fondaparinux 2.5 mg or placebo for the next 19–31 days. The primary end point of DVT, PE, or both occurred in 1.4% in the fondaparinux group versus 35% in the placebo group—a relative risk reduction of 95.9% ($P < 0.001$). Although there was a trend toward increased major bleeding in the fondaparinux group, there were no differences in the incidence of clinically relevant bleeding. The ACCP Guidelines for Prevention of VTE recommend that thromboprophylaxis be extended in the outpatient period for up to 35 days from the day of surgery [33]. Options for outpatient VTE prophylaxis include fondaparinux, LMWH, or warfarin. It is important to remember that symptomatic VTE events most commonly present after hospital discharge.

With respect to inferior vena cava (IVC) filters, the ACCP Guidelines for Prevention of VTE recommend against their use in hip fracture patients, even in situations when anticoagulant prophylaxis is contraindicated. It should be noted this is a weak recommendation given the lack of literature in this area. The ACCP Guidelines also recommend against routine Doppler (or duplex) ultrasound screening for DVT in asymptomatic hip fracture patients prior to hospital discharge.

Delirium

Delirium, defined as an acute disorder of attention and cognition, is commonly encountered in elderly hospitalized patients. Hip fracture patients have shown to be a very high risk population (incidence ranging from 9.5% to 61%), with the peak prevalence between postoperative days 2 and 5 [38–41]. Significant risk factors for delirium in hip fracture patients include advanced age, prior cognitive impairment/dementia, depression, low body mass index, fasting more than 12 hours, abnormal preoperative sodium level, and polypharmacy. A prospective study of 571 hip fracture patients was only able to identify a definite cause of delirium in 7% of cases, whereas 61% of cases were considered multifactorial [40]. One study found that delirium caused a nearly fourfold longer length of hospital stay for hip fracture patients [39], while another study reported compromised ambulation at time of discharge and at 6 months after surgery [41].

Efforts to prevent delirium in patients hospitalized for hip surgery have been studied using pharmacological and nonpharmacological strategies. Proactive geriatric consultation as a means of reducing delirium after hip fracture surgery was studied in a prospective, randomized, blinded trial of 126 patients aged 65 and older [42]. The intervention group received daily visits from a geriatrician who made targeted recommendations based on a structured protocol. Delirium was diagnosed in 32% of the intervention group versus 50% in those receiving "usual care," representing a risk reduction of more than 33% ($P = 0.04$). Severe delirium was reduced by an even greater margin. A similar but more recent prospective intervention study also reported a significant reduction in delirium in elderly hip fracture patients; 34% in the control group versus 22% in the intervention group, a 35% reduction ($P = 0.031$) [43]. Common interventions included daily screening for delirium, supplemental oxygen, IV fluids for hydration when fasting, adequate pain relief, and avoidance of polypharmacy. A detailed discussion of delirium can be found in Chapter 12.

Urinary Tract Infections and Bladder Management

Urinary tract infections (UTI) are commonly diagnosed in patients with chronic debility and immobility, including hip fracture patients. Johnstone et al. prospectively studied 88 hip fracture patients with urine cultures at the time of surgery and 48 hours postoperatively [44]. Of all patients, 12.5% had positive urine cultures at the time of surgery, whereas 42% had a positive culture at 48 hours postoperatively. Intracapsular fractures, advanced age, and surgical delay of more than 48 hours were all significant predictors of having a postoperative UTI. It should be noted, however, that data are extremely limited with respect to management of bacteriuria for joint replacement patients. Orthopedic surgeons tend to fear the possibility of prosthetic joint infection and prefer to treat patients with asymptomatic bacteriuria. Although there is no data to contradict this practice, one must be aware of the many risks of unnecessary antibiotic use, particularly in the higher-risk elderly population.

The extended use of indwelling urinary catheters beyond the immediate postoperative period is associated with decreased likelihood of discharge to home, rehospitalization for UTI and sepsis, and 30-day mortality in hip fracture patients [45]. Studies have compared the short-term use of indwelling urinary catheters versus intermittent catheterization postoperatively in joint replacement [46] and hip fracture patients [47], and have both been shown to reduce the incidence of urinary retention, an important risk factor for symptomatic UTI. A commonly accepted practice in this patient population is to use an indwelling catheter with removal on the first postoperative day.

Pressure Ulcers

Pressure ulcers represent a significant problem for hospitalized patients and can lead to increased risk of pain, infection, and prolonged hospitalization.

The incidence of pressure ulcers in hip fracture patients ranges from 10% to 40% [48]. An analysis of a retrospective cohort study that included 9400 elderly patients hospitalized for hip fracture surgery found that after adjusting for confounding variables, the factors associated with an increased risk for hospital-acquired pressure ulcers included the following: longer wait before surgery, ICU stay, longer length of surgery, and receipt of general anesthesia [49]. Special mattresses have been shown to reduce the risk of hospital-acquired pressure ulcers in hip fracture patients [50]. A prospective study involving six European countries identified several statistically significant risk factors associated with pressure ulcers at time of discharge, including age ≥71, dehydration, nutrition status, and sensory perception deficits [51]. This study also found that hip fracture patients with diabetes were at increased risk for developing pressure ulcers. A detailed discussion about pressure ulcers can be found in Chapter 11.

Pain Management

Despite the critical importance of adequate pain control among patients with hip fracture, there is little evidence to support a specific pain management strategy. A recent systematic review included 83 studies that addressed many pain management modalities, including nerve blockade, spinal anesthesia, systemic analgesia, traction, neurostimulation, and complementary/alternative medicine [52]. The authors found moderate evidence to suggest that nerve blockades are effective for relieving acute pain and reducing delirium. This review also found that traction was not an effective measure for pain control, and there was insufficient evidence on the benefits and harms of the other interventions. Despite the common use of systemic analgesics (i.e., opioids and nonsteroidal anti-inflammatory drugs), there was inadequate data to endorse firm conclusions about their effectiveness among hip fracture patients.

In clinical practice, prescribing opioids is a reasonable approach to manage pain associated with hip fracture. In the immediate perioperative period, this can be achieved via patient-controlled analgesia administration with conversion to an oral regimen on the first postoperative day. Judicious use of opioids is important given their deliriogenic tendencies; however, it is important to realize that pain itself is also a risk factor for delirium. Adjunctive therapies for pain control, such as acetaminophen, nonsteroidal anti-inflammatory drugs, and ice, are other options commonly employed. It may be appropriate to schedule pain medications for patients who are less willing or able to request them when needed. This strategy can prevent pain from becoming severe and more difficult to manage.

Although constipation is a common postoperative problem, hip fracture patients are at particularly high risk as they are typically older, with limited mobility, and commonly exposed to opioids for pain control. There is a scarcity of data regarding the use of laxatives to prevent constipation in orthopedic surgery patients on opioids. However, prescribing scheduled stool softeners and laxatives as a preventive measure in hip fracture patients is sensible in most cases. Promoting adequate hydration, prompt postoperative nutritional intake, and early mobilization are also practical measures that may reduce the risk of constipation.

Anemia

Perioperative blood loss is common after major surgery, with hip fracture surgery being no exception. As anemia is a relatively frequent diagnosis in the elderly population, such blood loss can often lead to levels of hemoglobin that prompt consideration of packed red blood cell transfusion. A prospective study of 546 patients aimed to determine the total blood loss associated with hip fracture surgery [53]. Although the observed intraoperative blood loss ranged from 200 to 500 mL depending on the type of hip surgery performed, the hidden blood loss (calculated from hemoglobin levels and estimated blood volume according to gender, body mass, and height) was an additional 1000–1500 mL. The authors also showed that this "hidden" blood loss was significantly associated with medical complications and an increased hospital stay. The authors concluded that total blood loss after hip fracture surgery is much greater than that observed intraoperatively and that close monitoring of postoperative hemoglobin may be necessary to detect and avoid anemia.

The threshold for postoperative blood transfusion is controversial, with limited data to guide management. A recent randomized controlled trial sought to determine if a liberal strategy of blood transfusion improves functional recovery and reduces morbidity and mortality among postoperative hip fracture patients with cardiovascular disease or risk factors for cardiovascular disease [54]. A total of 2016 patients (average age 81.6 years) were randomized to either a liberal transfusion strategy (to maintain a hemoglobin of 10 grams/deciliter or higher) or a restrictive transfusion strategy (for symptoms of anemia or for a hemoglobin of <8 g/dL at the discretion of the physician). The primary endpoint was death or an inability to walk across a room without human assistance on 60-day follow-up. The results showed no difference in the primary end point between the two groups, nor any difference in other measures, including acute coronary syndrome, stroke, hospital length of stay, or other functional measures. Given these results, it seems reasonable to withhold red-cell transfusions in the absence of symptoms of anemia or a hemoglobin >8 g/dL.

Physical and Occupational Therapy

The multidisciplinary team caring for hip fracture patients must also include physical and occupational therapists. Several factors can greatly increase the immobility of hip fracture patients, including delays awaiting surgery, pain, fatigue, deconditioning, and postoperative complications. Siu et al. conducted a prospective cohort study of 532 hip fracture patients to determine if the number of days of immobility correlated with functional status and survival [55]. The investigators observed that patients who were immobile for longer had worse functional outcomes at 2 months and higher mortality at 6 months. Thus, early assisted ambulation is associated with accelerated functional recovery and is an important component of postoperative care for hip fracture patients.

Intensive physical therapy (PT) also appears to be beneficial for recovery. A recent randomized controlled trial compared standard PT (30 minutes per day of supervised PT in the hospital with no home PT) to intensive PT (60 minutes per day of supervised PT in the hospital in addition to an unsupervised home program) [56]. One year following hip fracture surgery, patients who received the intensive PT had a significantly decreased rate of falls by 25%.

Approximately half of hip fracture patients are discharged to a skilled nursing facility after the acute hospitalization [3]. This is not surprising, as this patient population is typically elderly, frail, and requires goal directed physical and occupational therapy in order to return to their prefracture level of function. For many patients, the need for a skilled nursing facility is apparent very early in the hospitalization. The discharge planning process, with involvement of the social worker and/or discharge planner, should be initiated at the time of admission to optimize hospital throughput and avoid discharge delays. A detailed discussion of the discharge process can be found in Chapter 13.

Osteoporosis

Another consideration for hospitalists while caring for hip fracture patients is osteoporosis prevention and treatment. The National Osteoporosis Foundation (NOF) considers that postmenopausal women and men over the age of 50 with a hip fracture are candidates for osteoporosis treatment [57]. Recommendations include calcium and vitamin D supplementation with regular weight-bearing, muscle-strengthening, and balance-training exercises. Although the published data are not fully consistent, meta-analyses suggest that calcium supplementation of at least 1200 mg/d [58] and vitamin D supplementation of 800 IU/d [59] may decrease fracture risk in those over 50 years of age. These dosages are also consistent with recommendations from the American Association of Clinical Endocrinologists Osteoporosis Task Force and the NOF. Although calcium and vitamin D supplementation are effective and low-risk interventions, consistent administration for hip fracture patients is poor. In an observational cohort study using a large database involving 318 U.S. hospitals and 51,346 patients aged 65 years or greater, Jennings et al. examined in-hospital treatment with calcium and vitamin D for patients hospitalized for hip fracture [60]. Only 6.6% of patients received calcium and vitamin D at any time after surgery. The authors concluded that the in-hospital initiation of osteoporosis treatment for hip fracture patients is an opportunity to improve patient care.

Bisphosphonates are another therapy of interest for the hip fracture population. A yearly intravenous infusion of zoledronic acid was compared with placebo in a randomized, double-blind trial of 2127 patients who suffered a low-trauma hip fracture within 90 days [61]. All patients received calcium and vitamin D supplementation, and the primary end point was a new clinical fracture. The authors reported a statistically significant 35% risk reduction in new fractures in patients who received zoledronic acid, as well as a reduction in all-cause mortality. A more recent study used prospectively collected data from a previous randomized trial of osteoporosis quality improvement for hip fracture patients to determine the effect of oral bisphosphonate therapy on fracture risk and mortality [62]. Exposure to bisphosphonate therapy was independently associated with reduced mortality, as well as the composite endpoint of death or fracture. Although further studies may be needed, initiation of bisphosphonate therapy may prove to be a worthwhile intervention for hospitalists to employ for hip fracture patients during hospitalization or upon hospital discharge.

Quality Improvement Measures

The Surgical Care Improvement Project (SCIP) [63] is a national patient safety campaign that began in 2005 with the goal to reduce surgical morbidity and mortality through collaborative efforts. SCIP is sponsored by the Centers for Medicare and Medicaid Services (CMS) and includes a national quality partnership with several organizations, including the Joint Commission. The SCIP measures associated with hip fracture patients (who undergo hip arthroplasty) include the following:

- Appropriate VTE prophylaxis started within 24 hours
- Appropriate antibiotics for surgical site infection prophylaxis started within 1 hour before incision and discontinued within 24 hours
- Urinary catheter removal on postoperative day 1 or 2.

At the writing of this chapter, hospital participation is voluntary for these data collection efforts. However, CMS currently reduces hospital reimbursement if they do not report their performance on these measures.

In summary, hip fractures are a potentially devastating injury with a high rate of morbidity and mortality. Hospitalists are poised to provide effective, evidence-based care for this high-risk, medically complicated population as part of the multidisciplinary team. Hospitalists have demonstrated improved perioperative outcomes for hip fracture patients, including less hospital complications and a reduced length of stay. Postoperative complications are not uncommon in hip fracture patients, with cardiovascular, pulmonary, delirium, VTE, anemia, and pressure ulcers being the most common. Hospitalists need to be aware of the patient's individual risk of developing complications and how to implement appropriate risk reductions strategies. Box 9.1 summarizes some of the key hospitalist interventions in the care of a hip fracture patient.

REFERENCES

1. Zuckerman JD. Hip fracture. *N Engl J Med* 1996;334:1519–1525.
2. Barsoum WK, Helfand R, Krebs V, Whinney C. Managing perioperative risk in the hip fracture patient. *Cleve Clin J Med* 2006;73(Suppl. 1):S46–S50.
3. Brauer CA, Coca-Perraillon M, Cutler DM, Rosen AB. Incidence and mortality of hip fractures in the United States. *JAMA* 2009;302:1573–1579.
4. Magaziner J, Hawkes W, Hebel JR, et al. Recovery from hip fracture in eight areas of function. *J Gerontol A Biol Sci Med Sci* 2000;55:M498–M507.
5. Kirkland LL, Kashiwagi DT, Burton C, Cha S, Varkey P. The Charlson Comorbidity Index score as a predictor of 30-day mortality after hip fracture surgery. *Am J Med Qual* 2011;26:461–467.
6. Targownik LE, Lix LM, Metge CJ, Prior HJ, Leung S, Leslie WD. Use of proton pump inhibitors and risk of osteoporosis-related fractures. *CMAJ* 2008;179:319–326.
7. Ngamruengphong S, Leontiadis GI, Radhi S, Dentino A, Nugent K. Proton pump inhibitors and risk of fracture: A systematic review and meta-analysis of observational studies. *Am J Gastroenterol* 2011;106:1209–1218.
8. Gillespie WJ, Gillespie LD, Parker MJ. Hip protectors for preventing hip fractures in older people. *Cochrane Database Syst Rev* 2010;(10):CD001255.
9. Phy MP, Vanness DJ, Melton LJ, 3rd, et al. Effects of a hospital model on elderly patients with hip fracture. *Arch Intern Med* 2005;165:796–801.

10. Batsis JA, Phy MP, Melton LJ, 3rd, et al. Effects of a hospitalist care model on mortality of elderly patients with hip fractures. *J Hosp Med* 2007;2:219–225.

11. Roy A, Heckman MG, Roy V. Associations between the hospitalist model of care and quality-of-care-related outcomes in patients undergoing hip fracture surgery. *Mayo Clin Proc* 2006;81:28–31.

12. Friedman SM, Mendelson DA, Bingham KW, Kates SL. Impact of a comanaged geriatric fracture center on short-term hip fracture outcomes. *Arch Intern Med* 2009;169:1712–1717.

13. Grimes JP, Gregory PM, Noveck H, et al. The effects of time-to-surgery on mortality and morbidity in patients following hip fracture. *Am J Med* 2002;112:702–709.

14. Orosz GM, Magaziner J, Hannan EL, et al. Association of timing of surgery for hip fracture and patient outcomes. *JAMA* 2004;291:1738–1743.

15. Al-Ani AN, Samuelsson B, Tidermark J, et al. Early operation on patients with a hip fracture improved the ability to return to independent living. *J Bone Joint Surg Am* 2008;90:1436–1442.

16. Gdalevich M, Cohen D, Yosef D, Tauber C. Morbidity and mortality after hip fracture: The impact of operative delay. *Arch Orthop Trauma Surg* 2004;124:334–340.

17. Bottle A, Aylin P. Mortality associated with delay in operation after hip fracture: Observational study. *BMJ* 2006;332:947–951.

18. Morrison RS, Chassin MR, Siu AL. The medical consultant's role in caring for patients with hip fracture. *Ann Intern Med* 1998;128:1010–1020.

19. Shiga T, Wajima Z, Ohe Y. Is operative delay associated with increased mortality of hip fracture patients? Systematic review, meta-analysis, and meta-regression. *Can J Anaesth* 2008;55:146–154.

20. Simunovic N, Devereaux PJ, Sprague S, et al. Effect of eary surgery after hip fracture on mortality and complications: Systematic review and meta-analysis. *CMAJ* 2010;182:1609–1616.

21. Vidan MT, Sanchez E, Gracia Y, Maranon E, Vaquero J, Serra JA. Causes and effects of surgical delay in patients with hip fracture. *Ann Intern Med* 2011;155:226–233.

22. Grant PJ, Wesorick DH. Perioperative medicine for the hospitalized patient. *Med Clin North Am* 2008;92:325–348.

23. Lee TH, Marcantonio ER, Mangione CM, et al. Derivation and prospective validation of a simple index for prediction of cardiac risk of major noncardiac surgery. *Circulation* 1999;100:1043–1049.

24. Fleisher LA, Beckman JA, Brown KA, et al. 2009 ACCF/AHA focused update on perioperative beta blockade incorporated into the ACC/AHA 2007 guidelines on perioperative cardiovascular evaluation and care for noncardiac surgery: A report of the American College of Cardiology Foundation/American Heart Association Task Force on Practice Guidelines. *J Am Coll Cardiol* 2009;54:e13–e118.

25. McFalls EO, Ward HB, Moritz TE, et al. Coronary-artery revascularization before elective major vascular surgery. *N Engl J Med* 2004;351:2795–2804.

26. Poldermans D, Schouten O, Vidakovic R, et al. A clinical randomized trial to evaluate the safety of a noninvasive approach in high-risk patients undergoing major vascular surgery. The DECREASE-V pilot study. *J Am Coll Cardiol* 2007;49:1763–1769.

27. Powers PJ, Gent M, Jay RM, et al. A randomized trial of less intense postoperative warfarin or aspirin therapy in the prevention of venous thromboembolism after surgery for fractured hip. *Arch Intern Med* 1989;149:771–774.

28. Agnelli G, Cosmi B, Di Filippo P, et al. A randomised, double-blind, placebo controlled trial of dermatan sulphate for prevention of deep vein thrombosis in hip fracture. *Thromb Haemost* 1992;67:203–208.

29. Lowe GD, Campbell AF, Meek DR, et al. Subcutaneous ancrod in prevention of deep-vein thrombosis after operation for fractured neck of femur. *Lancet* 1978;2:698–700.

30. Rogers PH, Walsh PN, MArder VJ, et al. Controlled trial of low-dose heparin and sulfinpyrazone to prevent venous thromboembolism after operation on the hip. *J Bone Joint Surg Am* 1978;60:758–762.

31. Todd CJ, Freeman CJ, Camilleri-Ferrante C, et al. Differences in mortality after fracture of the hip: The east Anglian audit. *BMJ* 1995;310:904–908.

32. Fisher CG, Blachut PA, Salvian AJ, et al. Effectiveness of pneumatic leg compression devices for the prevention of thromboembolic disease in orthopaedic trauma patients: A prospective, randomized study of compression alone versus no prophylaxis. *J Orthop Trauma* 1995;9:1–7.

33. Falck-Ytter Y, Francis CW, Johanson NA, et al. Prevention of VTE in orthopedic surgery patients. Antithrombotic therapy and prevention of thrombosis, 9th ed: American College of Chest Physicians evidence-based clinical practice guidelines. *Chest* 2012;141(2 Suppl.):e278S–e325S.

34. PEP Trial Collaborative Group. Prevention of pulmonary embolism and deep vein thrombosis with low dose aspirin: Pulmonary Embolism Prevention (PEP) trial. *Lancet* 2000;355:1295–1302.

35. Hefley WF, Jr., Nelson CL, Puskarich-May CL. Effect of delayed admission to the hospital on the preoperative prevalence of deep-vein thrombosis associated with fractures about the hip. *J Bone Joint Surg Am* 1996;78:581–583.

36. Zahn HR, Skinner JA, Porteous MJ. The preoperative prevalence of deep vein thrombosis in patients with femoral neck fractures and delayed operation. *Injury* 1999;30:605–607.

37. Eriksson BI, Lassen MR. PENTasaccharide in HIp-FRActure Surgery Plus Investigators. Duration of prophylaxis against venous thromboembolism with fondaparinux after hip fracture surgery: A multicenter, randomized, placebo-controlled, double-blind study. *Arch Intern Med* 2003;163:1337–1342.

38. Galanakis P, Bickel H, Gradinger R, et al. Acute confusional state in the elderly following hip surgery: Incidence, risk factors and complications. *Int J Geriatr Psychiatry* 2001;16:349–355.

39. Berggren D, Gustafson Y, Eriksson B, et al. Postoperative confusion after anesthesia in elderly patients with femoral neck fractures. *Anesth Analg* 1987;66:497–504.

40. Brauer C, Morrison RA, Silberzweig SB, Siu AL. The cause of delirium in patients with hip fracture. *Arch Intern Med* 2000;160:1556–1860.

41. Gustafson Y, Berggren D, Brannstrom B, et al. Acute confusional states in elderly patients treated for femoral neck fracture. *J Am Geriatr Soc* 1988;36:525–530.

42. Marcantonio ER, Flacker JM, Wright RJ, Resnick NM. Reducing delirium after hip fracture: A randomized trial. *J Am Geriatr Soc* 2001;49:516–522.

43. Bjorkelund KB, Hommel A, Thorngren KG, Gustafson L, Larsson S, Lundberg D. Reducing delirium in elderly patients with hip fracture: A multi-factorial intervention study. *Acta Anaesthesiol Scand* 2010;54:678–688.

44. Johnstone DJ, Morgan NH, Wilkinson MC, Chissell HR. Urinary tract infection and hip fracture. *Injury* 1995;26:89–91.

45. Wald H, Epstein A, Kramer A. Extended use of indwelling urinary catheters in postoperative hip fracture patients. *Med Care* 2005;43:1009–1017.

46. Michelson JD, Lotke PA, Steinberg ME. Urinary-bladder management after total joint-replacement surgery. *N Engl J Med* 1988;319:321–326.

47. Skelly JM, Guyatt GH, Kalbfleisch R, et al. Management of urinary retention after surgical repair of hip fracture. *CMAJ* 1992;146:1185–1189.

48. Beaupre LA, Jones CA, Saunders LD, et al. Best practices for elderly hip fracture patients. A systematic overview of the evidence. *J Gen Intern Med* 2005;20:1019–1025.

49. Baumgarten M, Margolis D, Berlin JA, et al. Risk factors for pressure ulcers among elderly hip fracture patients. *Wound Repair Regen* 2003;11:96–103.

50. Hofman A, Geelkerken RH, Wille J, et al. Pressure sores and pressure-decreasing mattresses: Controlled clinical trial. *Lancet* 1994;343:568–571.

51. Lindholm C, Sterner E, Romanelli M, et al. Hip fracture and pressure ulcers—the Pan-European Pressure Ulcer Study—intrinsic and extrinsic risk factors. *Int Wound J* 2008;5: 315–328.

52. Abou-Setta AM, Beaupre LA, Rashiq S, et al. Comparative effectiveness of pain management interventions for hip fracture: A systematic review. *Ann Intern Med* 2011;155: 234–245.

53. Foss ND, Kehlet H. Hidden blood loss after surgery for hip fracture. *J Bone Joint Surg Br* 2006;88-B:1053–1059.

54. Carson JL, Terrin ML, Noveck H, et al. Liberal or restrictive transfusion in high-risk patients after hip surgery. *N Engl J Med* 2011;365:2453–2462.

55. Siu AL, Penrod JD, Boockvar KS, et al. Early ambulation after hip fracture; effects on function and mortality. *Arch Intern Med* 2006;166:766–771.

56. Bischoff-Ferrari HA, Dawson Hughes B, Platz A, et al. Effect of high-dosage cholcalciferol and extended physiotherapy on complications after hip fracture. *Arch Intern Med* 2010;170:813–820.

57. National Osteoporosis Foundation. *Clinician's Guide to Prevention and Treatment of Osteoporosis*. Washington, DC: National Osteoporosis Foundation, 2010.

58. Tang BM, Eslick GD, Nowson C, et al. Use of calcium or calcium in combination with vitamin D supplementation to prevent fractures and bone loss in people aged 50 years and older: A meta-analysis. *Lancet* 2007;370:657–666.

59. Bischoff-Ferrari HA, Willett WC, Wong JB, et al. Fracture prevention with vitamin D supplementation: A meta-analysis of randomized controlled trials. *JAMA* 2005;293: 2257–2264.

60. Jennings LA, Auerbach AD, Maselli J, Pekow PS, Lindenauer PK, Lee SJ. Missed opportunities for osteoporosis treatment in patients hospitalized for hip fracture. *J Am Geriatr Soc* 2010;58:650–657.

61. Lyles KW, Colon-Emeric CS, Magaziner JS, et al. Zoledronic acid and clinical fractures and mortality after hip fractures. *N Engl J Med* 2007;357:1799–1809.

62. Beaupre LA, Morrish DW, Hanley DA, et al. Oral bisphosphonates are associated with reduced mortality after hip fracture. *Osteoporos Int* 2011;22:983–991.

63. The Joint Commission. Surgical Care Improvement Project. 2012. Available at: http://www.jointcommission.org/surgical_care_improvement_project/ (accessed April 11, 2013).

CHAPTER 10

FALLS AND MOBILITY DURING HOSPITALIZATION

Cynthia J. Brown
Donna M. Bearden

HOSPITAL FALLS

Among older adults, hospital-related falls are common, costly, and associated with adverse outcomes, including fractures, head injury, and even death. In 2008, the Centers for Medicare and Medicaid Services (CMS) identified falls with injury as a preventable or "never" event and as such will not fund the treatment of any complications relating to the fall. While the reduction in Medicare payments to hospitals is estimated to be less than 0.01% nationally [1], there has been a significant focus by hospitals on reducing falls, at times to the detriment of patient mobility. Because guidelines for fall prevention in the hospital setting have yet to be developed, hospitals have produced their own fall prevention measures to address pay for performance initiatives. While the emphasis on patient safety is important and necessary, CMS might serve the older adult population better by rewarding hospitals for safe mobility, not just the prevention of falls [2].

Falls Tracking and Reporting

In most hospitals, an incident reporting system is used to document patient falls, circumstances, and any injury sustained due to the fall. Rates are calculated based on the number of falls per 1000 patient days, allowing small and large hospitals to compare their rates. Currently, more than 1500 hospital systems report their falls data to the National Database of Nursing Quality Indicators (NDNQI). This national proprietary database of the American Nurses Association collects and evaluates nurse-sensitive data and provides

Hospitalists' Guide to the Care of Older Patients, Edited by Brent C. Williams, Preeti N. Malani, and David H. Wesorick.

participating hospitals with confidential comparison data based on unit type. Comparison data based on hospital groups, including the number of staffed beds or teaching status, can also be provided. Data from NDNQI can be used for patient safety and quality improvement initiatives, as well as to satisfy reporting requirements for Joint Commission, CMS, or the Magnet Hospital program. The Magnet Recognition Program® was developed by the American Nurses Credentialing Center (ANCC) and recognizes healthcare organizations for quality patient care, nursing excellence, and innovations in professional nursing practice [3]. The Hospital Inpatient Quality Reporting (Hospital IQR) program originally mandated by the 2003 Medicare Prescription Drug, Improvement, and Modernization Act (MMA) of 2003 allows CMS to pay hospitals that report specific quality measures a higher annual update to their payment rates [4]. This program also provides CMS with hospital quality of care data that is available to consumers through the Hospital Compare website at http://www.hospitalcompare.hhs.gov [5].

Risk Factors for Falls During Hospitalization

As with other geriatric syndromes, falls in older adults are usually multifactorial in nature. Risk factors unique to the individual, often termed intrinsic risk factors, as well as factors unique to the hospital environment, often termed extrinsic factors, can contribute to the fall risk of older hospitalized patients. In addition, while identifying individual risk factors is important, the interaction of all of the patient's risk factors is also critically important. Among community-dwelling older adults, the percentage of persons falling increased from 27% for those with one or fewer risk factors to 78% for those with four or more [6]. While assessing an individual patient's fall risk is an appropriate role for the hospitalist, the clinician may also need to consider if extrinsic factors are contributing to patient falls and if so, consider advocating for environmental changes to reduce fall risk. A review of the literature reveals, however, that individual risk factors for falling contribute significantly more to the patient's fall risk than environmental factors in the hospital.

Intrinsic Risk Factors: On Admission

All hospitalized older patients should be considered at risk for falling. Chronic disease states unique to the individual contribute to fall risk, as well as acute illnesses that may have resulted in their current hospitalization. If possible, asking the patient or family member if the patient has fallen in the past year, or if the current admission was associated with a fall, may help to identify those patients at even higher risk than others.

The initial patient history on admission or transfer should include a thorough review of the patient's medications. Psychotropic medication use has consistently been shown to put older adults at increased risk of falling in any setting. Benzodiazepines and opiates are perhaps the most common offending agents, but antidepressants, antipsychotics and sedative hypnotics, as well as sleeping aids, also contribute to fall risk. According to the most recent Geriatric Review Syllabus, the risk of falls increases in older adults taking more than one psychotropic medication, and among older adults taking more than three or four medications of any type [7]. Other medications associated with increased risk of falling in the older adult include hypoglycemic agents, digoxin, diuretics, and type I antiarrythmic agents.

In addition to a thorough medication history, the patient's past medical history should be used to identify risk factors for falls. Older patients should be asked if they have a history of arthritis, such as osteoarthritis of the hips or knees, or rheumatoid arthritis, which can limit their mobility. Most neurological conditions can contribute to fall risk and should be specifically asked about. This includes questioning about peripheral neuropathies, Parkinson's disease, and a history of stroke, all of which increase risk for falling.

On physical examination, screening for visual impairment and postural hypotension may help to identify patients at high risk for falling. Heart rate and rhythm disturbances can increase risk as well. If identified, cognitive impairment and gait abnormalities can be precursors to falls.

Intrinsic Risk Factors: In the Hospital

Either on presentation to the hospital or after admission, many older adults develop additional problems that can lead to falls. As a result of their acute illness, they may be experiencing delirium on admission or develop this condition after being hospitalized. Falls in the hospital are also frequently associated with the need to toilet. Older adults with urinary incontinence, who may be receiving diuretics requiring frequent trips to the toilet may experience a fall. Likewise, those undergoing bowel preparations for gastrointestinal procedures may be at higher risk. Finally, many older adults in the hospital are recovering from procedures, and the pain and decreased mobility resulting from such procedures may result in a fall.

Extrinsic Risk Factors: In the Hospital

The traditional hospital environment can be very difficult for many older adults to navigate and can increase their risk for falls and injury. Institutional factors often cited as potential contributors to fall risk include rooms and halls with slick, hard floors, areas of low lighting and unstable furniture. In one study, transfers in and out of bed were identified as the cause of 42% of inpatient falls. Environmental faults identified included slippery floors, inappropriate door openings, poor placement of rails and accessories, and incorrect toilet and furniture heights [8]. A systematic review of randomized controlled trials of fall prevention interventions and subsequent meta-analysis found no convincing evidence for the isolated effectiveness of environmental modification programs [9], although these modifications have been a part of several multifactorial interventions.

Increased patient to nurse/staff ratio has also been shown to consistently place patients at increased risk for falling [10]. Falls tend to occur among new admissions to the hospital; most are not witnessed, and 50–70% occur from the bed, bedside chair, or while transferring between the two [11]. According to Ulrich, most evidence suggests that bedrails are ineffective for reducing the incidence of falls [12]. While bedrails have not been shown to reduce fall rate, they can be helpful for patients who have limited bed mobility. Unfortunately, despite weak methodological quality of evidence, the literature has raised significant concerns about bedrails leading to serious injuries when patients become entrapped, or climb over and fall from a greater height. The injuries reported in the literature and in case law appear to be more related to incorrect use as opposed to an inherent problem with the bed rails [13]. Individual assessment of the need for bed rails to promote both mobility and safety is necessary.

In several systematic reviews, six risk factor categories have emerged as significant despite the heterogeneity of the settings, populations, and risk factors studied. Given the lack of current guidelines, it is reasonable to focus fall prevention efforts on the most common modifiable risk factors [11] (Table 10.1).

Interventions

Because hospital falls are common and costly, the search for effective interventions to reduce falls and fall-related injuries has been intense for many

TABLE 10.1 Consistently Identified Risk Factors for Hospital Falls [11]

- History of recent fall
- Muscle weakness
- Behavioral disturbance, agitation or confusion
- Urinary incontinence or frequency
- Prescription of "culprit" medications including benzodiazepines, sedatives/hypnotics
- Postural hypotension or syncope.

years. Most hospitals employ "Universal Fall Precautions," which include procedures like assuring the hospital bed is locked and in its lowest position. To date, large literature reviews and meta-analyses have not found convincing evidence that single or multifactorial intervention fall reduction programs are beneficial. However, individual studies that have targeted patients' most important risk factors for falls have had some success in reducing fall rates.

Among single intervention programs to reduce fall risk, only the subacute settings tested supervised exercise programs as a means of reducing falls. Pooled data from three studies showed a significant reduction in the number of falls, although exercise programs may not be feasible in the acute care setting [14]. Other single interventions not shown to demonstrate benefit in the acute hospital setting included fall alert bracelets and vitamin D supplementation [11]. Evidence regarding the use of bed or chair alarms to reduce falls has been equivocal. A 12-month uncontrolled before-and-after study by Sahota demonstrated a significant reduction in the odds of being a faller among patients after hip fracture when bed alarms were used, although no significant reduction in fall rate was seen overall [15]. However, Shorr et al. found no differences in fall rates, relative risk of being a faller or percentage of patients subjected to physical restraint in an 18-month cluster randomized trial using such alarms [11, 16]. One study suggested that patients were more likely to fall on carpeted flooring than vinyl flooring and additional studies of flooring are ongoing [17].

Beds capable of being lowered to within inches of the floor have also been proposed as both a fall and an injury prevention measure. It has been postulated that if a patient falls from the "low bed," they will be less likely to injure themselves due to the relatively short distance they fall before impacting the ground. In addition, it is harder to get up from the low position, making it more likely staff will have time to intervene when a patient is trying to get out of bed unassisted. There has been a single cluster randomized trial of low height beds that included 22,036 participants and found no significant reduction in frequency of patient injuries due to the beds. However, this study also reported no injuries among either the control or the intervention groups. Further work is needed in this area to determine the impact of low height beds to reduce falls and injuries [18].

In the most recent Cochrane Collaboration systematic review on interventions to reduce falls in older people in nursing care facilities and hospitals, researchers examined single intervention programs and multifactorial interventions in the hospital setting [14]. Of the eleven randomized controlled trials in hospital settings, however, only one was in an acute hospital setting, six were in subacute settings, and four were in both acute and subacute care settings, making generalizability an issue. The reviewers found for patients who are in the hospital for more than a few weeks, multifactorial interventions reduced the rate of falls by 31% and the risk of falling by 27%. However, in the one study done in the acute care setting, no difference was seen in fall rate or risk of falling. In an earlier systematic review and meta-analysis, the authors noted a tendency towards a reduction in falls among the individual studies that targeted a patient's most important risk factors. However, to date, there is no conclusive evidence that hospital fall prevention programs can reduce falls.

Electronic health records and information technology holds some promise in achieving a goal of fall reduction. In a recently published cluster randomized control trial, investigators used health information technology to develop a fall prevention tool kit designed to reduce patient falls in acute care hospitals [19]. The toolkit linked the patient's risk factors, as documented on a fall risk assessment tool, to interventions to address those risk factors. This included tailored patient and family education materials, as well as an individualized fall prevention plan. The study compared patient fall rates and fall related injuries in four urban US hospitals on units that received either usual care or the intervention. They concluded that the fall prevention tool kit significantly reduced the rate of falls in the intervention group, particularly in patients aged 65 years and older. No significant effect was demonstrated in fall related injuries.

While the ideal approach to fall reduction and injury prevention remains to be elucidated, Oliver et al. argue for a best practice approach for preventing hospital falls, which might include four key components [11].

1. Implementation of a safer environment of care for all hospital inpatients
2. Identification of a patient's modifiable risk factors
3. Implementation of interventions to target those modifiable risk factors
4. Interventions to reduce the risk of injury or harm to those patients who do fall.

The American Geriatric Society suggests that a practical approach for physicians treating older adults at risk for falling includes targeting risk factors in three major domains: medication-related, mobility-related, and medical factors [7]. Table 10.2 describes risk factors in each of these three domains and provides potential interventions to reduce the risk of falls associated with these factors. For example, benzodiazepines are often used to promote sleep during hospitalization. However, these medications are associated with a higher risk of falls among persons who take them. Instead, nonpharmacological measures, such as control of nighttime environment (e.g. comfortable temperature, quiet, dark), limiting liquids in the evening

TABLE 10.2   Common Hospital Risk Factors and Potential Interventions

Risk factor	Potential intervention
Medication-related factors	
Use of benzodiazepines, sedative-hypnotics, antidepressants, or antipsychotics	Consider medications with less risk for falls. Taper dosage and discontinue medications, as able. Address sleep and mood problems with nonpharmacological interventions.
Recent change in dosage or number of prescription medications	Review medications and monitor response to dosage changes.
Mobility-related factors	
Presence of environmental hazards (poor lighting, cluttered pathways, slippery floors).	Improve lighting. Assure clear pathway to bathroom/toilet. Encourage every person who enters room to check for possible hazards, like spilled water, and correct or remove hazards quickly. Assure functional and correctly placed grab bars in bathrooms.
Presence of medical devices that limit safe mobility (intravenous lines, urinary catheters, oxygen).	Frequently reassess need for medical devices.
Impaired lower extremity strength, impaired gait or balance.	Physical therapy. Encourage patient to be out of bed with help. Prescribe and/or provide necessary ambulatory devices for safe mobility.
Medical factors	
Postural hypotension: drop in systolic blood pressure >20 mmHg (or >20%) with or without symptoms, within 3 minutes of position change from lying to standing.	Review medications for potential contributors and adjust dose as able, especially vasodilators and diuretics. Educate patient to change positions slowly. Encourage patient to sit up in bed or chair.
Specific diseases or symptoms associated with falling: Parkinson's disease, osteoarthritis, impaired cognition (dementia and delirium), urinary incontinence or frequency, carotid hypersensitivity, arrhythmias, and visual impairment.	Optimize medical therapy. Monitor for disease progression and impact on mobility and functional impairments Evaluate need for assistive devices. Consider bedside commode if frequent nighttime urination. Toileting schedules. Cardiac pacing in patients with carotid hypersensitivity who experience falls due to syncope. Encourage use of glasses.

Adapted with permission from Reuben DB, Herr KA, Pacala JT, et al. *Geriatrics At Your Fingertips*, 14th ed. New York: The American Geriatrics Society, 2012; table 46, p. 105.

and avoiding caffeine after lunch may be helpful strategies. If after careful review, a hypnotic medication is determined to be necessary, selective shorter-acting nonbenzodiazepine hypnotics at the lowest effective dose can be used [20].

Postfall Follow-Up

A fall occurs when an individual comes to rest inadvertently on a lower level or on the floor. If a fall occurs while a patient is hospitalized, the hospitalist staff should be notified immediately. A history of events surrounding the fall should be obtained from the patient, staff, and others who may have witnessed the fall. Potential contributors to the fall should be sought and corrected if possible, and secondary preventive strategies should be considered. Potential contributors include those identified in the patient's initial or follow-up fall risk assessments and described under intrinsic factors. Less common contributors to fall risk in the elderly that the hospitalist may need to consider include carotid sinus hypersensitivity and visual impairment.

Once a history has been taken, the patient should undergo a targeted physical examination that includes a check for postural hypotension, heart rate abnormalities, and arrhythmias. After assessment, a laboratory evaluation and other testing may be considered, depending on the results of the history and physical. Radiographs of injured areas, as well as cranial imaging for patients sustaining head trauma, should be considered. After needed testing has been ordered, the patient's medications should be reassessed. Potential offending agents, such as psychotropic medications, should be stopped or at least minimized as much as possible. Some medications such as benzodiazepines or opiates cannot be stopped abruptly if the patient has been on them for an extended period, but in many cases, they can be tapered. According to Assessing Care of Vulnerable Elders (ACOVE) guidelines, if a vulnerable older adult falls while hospitalized, the presence or absence of prodromal symptoms should be documented within 24 hours, and the patient should undergo a medication review during this time period as well [21].

In addition to the above, all fall events involving an older hospitalized adult should be evaluated in a process called the *postfall huddle*. The assessment is usually conducted by nursing staff and administrators to review events and circumstances surrounding the fall to prevent a similar event from occurring in the future. It may be beneficial for physicians to participate in this huddle, but there are no guidelines in the literature to direct physician involvement. Likewise, there is nothing in the literature to suggest that risk managers need to be notified of a fall occurrence. Healthcare providers should refer to their individual institutional policies. In addition, Table 10.3 provides additional sources of information about falls and fall prevention.

TABLE 10.3   Available Resources for Fall Prevention Materials

- The United States Department of Veterans Affairs, National Center for Patient Safety 2004 Falls Toolkit. http://www.patientsafety.gov/SafetyTopics/fallstoolkit/index.html.
- The Joint Commission Patient Safety Goals. http://www.jointcommission.org/patientsafety/nationalpatientsafetygoals.
- Australian Commission on Safety and Quality in Healthcare. Preventing falls and harm from falls in older people: Best practice guidelines for Australian hospitals, 2009. http://www.safetyandquality.gov.au/publications/preventing-falls-and-harm-from-falls-in-older-people-best-practice-guidelines-for-australian-hospitals-2009/
- Patient Safety First. The "how to" guide to reducing harm from falls. http://www.patientsafetyfirst.nhs.uk.

Coding for Fall Risk Assessment and Management

Unfortunately, current procedural terminology (CPT) codes and International Classification of Diseases (ICD) codes do not contain fall risk assessment or management codes. Providers must instead use individual codes that identify the condition increasing the patient's risk for falling. This applies to the post fall assessment as well. Providers may also code injuries related to the fall, but as pointed out earlier, Medicare will consider codes related to post fall care and assessment as "never event" codes.

HOSPITAL MOBILITY

In an effort to reduce falls among older adults, hospital mobility may be compromised. Bed rest and low mobility, defined as bed or bed to chair mobility, is common and associated with adverse outcomes [22]. Physiological changes associated with bed rest begin within hours of becoming supine, including orthostatic intolerance, muscle atrophy, and deconditioning [23]. Kortebein and colleagues demonstrated a 6.3% loss (95% confidence interval (CI) −3.1 to −9.5) of lower extremity lean muscle mass when comparing before and after bed rest in a group of *healthy* older adults age ≥65 years [24].

Several recent studies have noted, on average, older adults spend more than 80% of their hospital stay lying in bed and less than 50 minutes a day standing or walking [25, 26]. This low level of mobility has been associated with adverse outcomes, including functional decline, need for new nursing home admission, and death, even after controlling for illness severity, having an ICU or CCU stay, and comorbidity [22]. While the average hospital length of stay for older patients is only 5.5 days, the bed rest and low mobility that

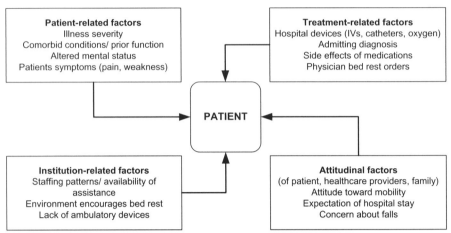

Figure 10.1   Perceived barriers to hospital mobility from the perspective of the patient, his or her nurse, and physician. This model of potential barriers to hospital mobility was developed based on qualitative interviews with patients, their nurses, and physicians. While some of the factors identified are not modifiable, others could be included as a component of an intervention to reduce both falls and low mobility (adapted from Brown CJ, et al. *J Hosp Med* 2009).

occurs even during that short time may lead to significant loss of lean muscle mass and may contribute to the functional decline observed at hospital discharge.

Barriers to Mobility

Unfortunately, the hospital environment is fraught with barriers to mobility. Several of the most commonly cited barriers are shown in Figure 10.1 [27]. While some of these barriers, such as illness severity and comorbidity, are not modifiable, others are clearly amendable and potential targets for improving the level of mobility older patients achieve.

Interventions to Improve Mobility

On admission, careful thought should be given to physician activity orders. Most patients do not require bed rest and progressive activity as patients recover from their medical illness may be highly beneficial. Indeed, research has revealed numerous medical conditions initially thought to require bed rest to reduce complications and improve recovery are actually improved

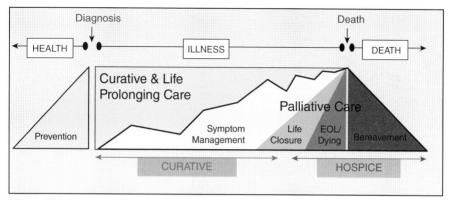

Figure 5.1 An integrated model of palliative care. This model of care emphasizes the coadministration of curative and palliative care across the spectrum of disease. Adapted from the World Health Organization Report on Cancer Pain and Palliative Care, reproduced with permission [4].

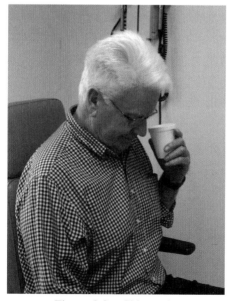

Figure 8.2   Chin tuck.

Hospitalists' Guide to the Care of Older Patients, Edited by Brent C. Williams, Preeti N. Malani, and David H. Wesorick.

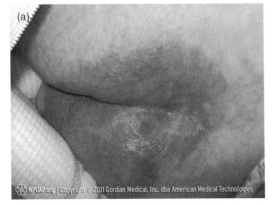

Treatment:

·turn and reposition every 2 hours

·moisture barrier cream *or* protective dressing, such as a hydrocolloid

·nursing to assess skin every shift

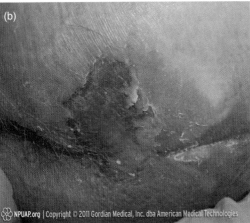

Treatment:

·turn and reposition every 2 hours

·moisture barrier cream *or* protective dressing such as a hydrocolloid or foam, if significant drainage (see table on dressings and indications)

·nursing to assess skin every shift

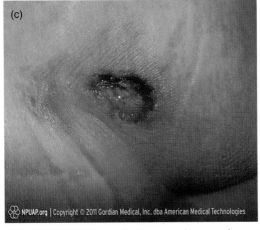

Treatment:

·turn and reposition every 2 hours

·moisture barrier cream to periwound

·dressing choice to wound based on tissue type and level of drainage (see table on dressings and indications)

·nursing to assess skin every shift

·assessment and maximization of nutrition

·level 1 matress (gel, foam, or static air overlay)

Figure 11.2   Stages of pressure ulcers and treatment plans. (a) Stage I: Nonblanchable erythema of intact skin. (b) Stage II: Partial thickness skin loss, no necrotic slough. (c) Stage III: Full thickness skin loss to the fascia, but not through the fascia. (d) Stage IV: Full thickness ulcer involving muscle, bone, or tendon. (e) Unstageable pressure ulcer. (f) Suspected deep tissue injury.

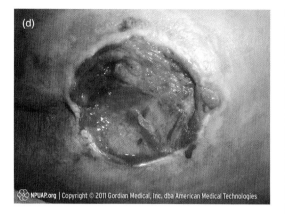

Treatment:

·turn and reposition every 2 hours

·moisture barrier cream to periwound

·dressing choice based on tissue
 type and level of drainage (see
 table on dressings and indications)

·nursing to assess skin every shift

·assessment and maximization
 of nutrition

·level 2 or 3 mattress (low air loss,
 alternating pressure, or high air loss);
 start with low air loss

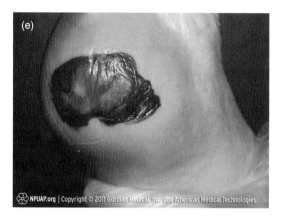

Treatment:

·turn and reposition every 2 hours

·dressing choice based on tissue
 type and level of drainage (see
 table on dressings and indications)

·nursing to assess skin every shift

·assessment and maximization of
 nutrition

·level 2 or 3 mattress if wound on
 trunk (low air loss, alternating
 pressure, or high air loss); start
 with low air loss

·debridement if slough or necrotic
 tissue is present

Figure 11.2 *(Continued)*

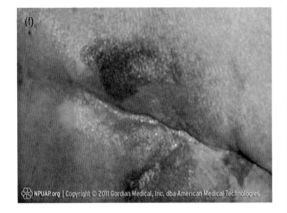

Treatment:

·turn and reposition every 2 hours

·when the skin begins to open, dressing choice based on tissue type and level of drainage (see table on dressings and indications)

·nursing to assess skin every shift

·assessment and maximization of nutrition

·because there is no break in skin, patient will not qualify for a specialty mattress under CMS guidelines. If the hospital owns its own pressure redistribution surfaces, the patient should be placed on it

·when the skin begins to open, debridement of necrotic tissue

Figure 11.2 *(Continued)*

with mobilization. For example, prior to the 1970s, patient admitted with a myocardial infarction were placed on bed rest for 6 weeks. Investigators realized that by reducing the length of bed rest, they improved mortality [28]. More recently, research has shown no significant difference between the frequency of new pulmonary embolus for patients with deep vein thrombosis treated with low molecular weight heparin and either kept on bed rest for 4–8 days or allowed to ambulate with compression bandages [29]. Importantly, patients who were allowed to ambulate had a faster reduction of pain and swelling initially, and were less likely to develop postthrombotic syndrome during the following few years [30].

Unfortunately, it is not enough to minimize bed rest orders. Active encouragement of safe mobility is critical. Patients need to be encouraged to sit up for meals and walk to the toilet with assistance as needed. Orders for physical therapy services can be helpful, but often therapists are only able to see patients once a day. To address this need for ambulatory assistance, several investigators have explored other potential options. In one randomized controlled trial, Mundy et al. used a nurse-driven protocol to increase ambulation among patients admitted with community-acquired pneumonia. They found patients in the progressive walking program were discharged home 1 day earlier than the control group without any increase in rehospitalization rate. This led to an average reduction in hospital costs of $1000 per patient [31]. In another small pilot study, transporters were used to walk with patients especially at night and on weekends. The study was shown to be feasible with patients receiving an average of 5.6 walks during the 2.4 days they were enrolled. However, no data is available as to improved outcomes at or after hospital discharge [32]. In a randomized controlled trial of a mobility intervention that included motivational interviewing and provision of assistance with ambulation twice a day, patients in the intervention group had improved community mobility 1 month after hospital discharge compared with the control group even after controlling for length of stay, comorbidity, and depression [33].

Other significant factors for both falls and limited mobility include patient symptoms, especially pain and weakness, hospital devices like intravenous lines and urinary catheters, medication side effects, and lack of ambulatory devices. Assessment of pain, the "fifth vital sign," and treatment of pain is obviously important for patient's well-being. While a patient may be at higher risk of falling due to pain medications, this should not be a reason to limit their pain relief. Healthcare providers also need to carefully weigh the risks and benefits of medical devices, like urinary catheters. In addition to being a conduit for infection, catheters can also significantly limit mobility and have been termed a "one-point restraint" [34]. It has been suggested that urinary catheters are used too frequently, especially among older adults with limited mobility, cognitive impairment, and risk for falls [35]. Lack of ambulatory devices is a common issue, with patients leaving their devices at home for fear of losing them. Yet if a patient walks with a walker at home, it is unreasonable to believe they will be safe to walk without an assistive device in the hospital. Either provision of loaner equipment or encouragement to have the ambulatory device brought from home is a reasonable option to encourage mobility and reduce falls.

Importantly, many of these perceived barriers to mobility are also considered risk factors for falls. There is significant tension between the goals of reducing falls and of maintaining mobility. However, the two goals are not mutually exclusive. Fisher et al. examined the association between ambulatory activity and falls and found patient falls were more likely to be associated with cognitive and hospital environmental issues than the actual time spent walking [36]. In the intensive care unit, an out of bed activity protocol was initiated after patients were deemed to be medically stable, even if they remained on the ventilator. The protocol included progressive activities twice daily, which included sitting on the side of the bed, with progression to transfers and ambulation. At discharge from intensive care, after participating in a graduated mobility protocol, 69% of patients were able to walk at least 100 ft. Six activity-related adverse events were defined, including fall to knees, nasogastric (NG) tube removal, systolic blood pressure >200 or <90 mm Hg, oxygen desaturation <80%, and extubation. Adverse events were infrequent, occurring in 14 of 1449 (0.96%) activity events, with falls and orthostatic hypotension being most common with 5 and 4 occurrences, respectively [37]. It is important for the healthcare team to balance the possible risk of a fall with the benefit seen through increased mobility, as shown in this intensive care unit study.

As additional proof, one structured fall prevention program included fall risk assessment, assistance with transfers and use of the toilet, provision of ambulatory devices as needed, and early mobilization strategies encouraging patients to get out of bed as early as possible. Using this protocol, there was an 18% reduction in falls in the intervention group [38]. The Hospital Elder Life Program (HELP) was initially developed to reduce the incidence of hospital delirium. However, the strategies recommended to prevent delirium are also being used to prevent falls, including scheduled toileting, provision of physical therapy, and early mobilization. Unpublished data from hospitals that use HELP reveal significant decreases in fall rates, which are not surprising as delirium and falls share common risk factors, such as cognitive and functional impairment and low mobility [2, 39].

In summary, strong evidence for effective hospital fall prevention programs is still lacking despite numerous studies. Multifactorial interventions that address modifiable risk factors appear most likely to succeed. However, it is imperative that healthcare providers and hospitals recognize the inherent tradeoff between safety, as measured by fall rate, and mobility. Falls may occur as a consequence of patients mobilizing when not closely supervised by hospital staff as they recover from their acute illness. It is reasonable to consider that there will be inevitable consequences of promoting rehabilitation and respecting patient autonomy. For patients with capacity, the balance between safety and rehabilitation is theirs to make. For patients who are dependent on staff or surrogates for decision-making, seeking a balance between the risk of harm from falls and the risk of harm from impaired independence is essential [11].

REFERENCES

1. Rosenthal MB. Nonpayment for performance? Medicare's new reimbursement rule. *N Engl J Med* 2007;357(16):1573–1575.
2. Inouye SK, Brown CJ, Tinetti ME. Medicare nonpayment, hospital falls and unintended consequences. *N Engl J Med* 2009;360(23):2390–2393.
3. American Nurses Credentialing Center. Announcing a new model for ANCC's Magnet Recognition Program. 2008. Available at: http://www.nursecredentialing.org/Magnet/ProgramOverview.aspx (accessed April 11, 2013).
4. National Database of Nursing Quality Indicators (NDNQI): Transforming data into quality care. 2010. Available at: http://nursingquality.org (accessed June 10, 2013).
5. Department of Health and Human Services (HHS). Hospital Compare. Available at: http://www.hospitalcompare.hhs.gov (accessed April 11, 2013).
6. MacCulloch PA, Gardner T, Bonner A. Comprehensive fall prevention programs across settings: A review of the literature. *Geriatr Nurs* 2007;28(5):306–311.
7. Berry SD, Kiel DP. Falls. In: Pacala JT, Sullivan GM (eds.), *Geriatrics Review Syllabus*, 7th ed. New York: American Geriatrics Society, 2010, pp. 250–260.
8. Brandis SA. collaborative Occupational therapy and nursing approach to falls prevention in hospital inpatients. *J Qual Clin Pract* 1999;19(4):215–221.
9. Chang JT, Morton SC, Rubenstein LZ, Mojica WA, et al. Interventions for the prevention of falls in older adults: Systematic review and meta-analysis of randomised clinical trials. *BMJ* 2004;328(7441):680.
10. Kraus MJ, Evanoff B, Hitcho E, Ngugi KE, et al. A Case-control study of patient, medication, and care-related risk factors for inpatient falls. *J Gen Intern Med* 2005;20:116–122.
11. Oliver D, Healey F, Haines TP. Preventing falls and fall-related injuries in hospitals. *Clin Geriatr Med* 2010;26:645–692.
12. Ulrich R, Quan X, Zimring C, Joseph A, et al. The role of the physical environment in the hospital of the 21st century: A once-in-a-lifetime opportunity. Report to the Center for Health Design. September 2004.
13. Healey F, Oliver D, Milne A, Connelly JB. The effect of bedrails on falls and injury: A systematic review of clinical studies. *Age Ageing* 2008;37:368–378.
14. Cameron ID, Murray GR, Gillespie LD, Robertson MC, et al. Interventions for preventing falls in older people in nursing care facilities and hospitals. *Cochrane Database Syst Rev* 2010;(1):CD005465.

15. Sahota O. Vitamin D and inpatient falls. *Age Ageing* 2009;38(3):339–340.

16. Shorr RI, Mion L, Rosenblatt L, et al. Ascertainment of patient falls in hospital using an evaluation service: Comparison with incident reports. *J Am Geriatr Soc* 2007;55 (Suppl. 4):S1–S246.

17. Donald IP, Pitt K, Armstron E, Shuttleworth H. Preventing falls on and elderly care rehabilitation ward. *Clin Rehabil* 2000;14(2):178–185.

18. Haines TP, Bell RAR, Varghese PN. Pragmatic, cluster radomized trial of a policy to introduce low-low beds to hospital wards for the prevention of falls and fall injuries. *J Am Geriatr Soc* 2010;58:435–441.

19. Dykes PC, Carroll DL, Hurley A, et al. Fall prevention in acute care hospitals. *JAMA* 2010;304(17):1912–1918.

20. Cohen-Zion M, Ancoli-Israel S. Sleep disorders. In: Halter JB, Ouslander JG, Tinetti ME, Studenski SA, High KP, Asthana S (eds.), *Hazzard's Geriatric Medicine and Gerontology*, 6th ed. New York: McGraw Hill Medical, 2009, pp. 678–680.

21. Arora VM, McGory ML, Fung CH. Quality indicators for hospitalization and surgery in vulnerable elders. *J Am Geriatr Soc* 2007;55:S347–S358.

22. Brown CJ, Friedkin RJ, Inouye SK. Prevalence and outcomes of low mobility in hospitalized older patients. *J Am Geriatr Soc* 2004;52(8):1263–1270.

23. Fortney SM, Schneider VS, Greenleaf JE. The physiology of bedrest. In: Fregly MJ, Blatteis CM (eds.), *Handbook of Physiology. Environmental Physiology*. Bethesda, MD: American Physiological Society, 1996, pp. 889–939.

24. Kortebein P, Ferrando A, Lombeida J, Wolfe R, Evans WJ. Effects of 10 days of bed rest on skeletal muscle in healthy older adults. *J Am Med Assoc* 2007;297:1772–1773.

25. Brown CJ, Redden D, Flood KL, Allman RM. The underrecognized epidemic of low mobility during hospitalization. *J Am Geriatr Soc* 2009;57:1660–1665.

26. Fisher SR, Graham JE, Brown CJ, et al. Factors that differentiate level of ambulation in hospitalization older adults. *Age Ageing* 2012;41(1):107–111.

27. Brown CJ, Williams BR, Woodby LL, Davis LL, Allman RM. Barriers to mobility during hospitalization from the perspectives of the older patients and their nurses and physicians. *J Hosp Med* 2007;2(5):305–313.

28. Harpur JE, Conner ET, Hamilton M, et al. Controlled trial of early mobilization and discharge from hospital in uncomplicated myocardial infarction. *Lancet* 1971;2: 1331–1334.

29. Aschwanden M, Labs KH, Engel H, et al. Acute deep vein thrombosis: Early mobilization does not increase the frequency of pulmonary embolism. *Thromb Haemost* 2001;85: 42–46.

30. Partsch H. Ambulation and compression after deep vein thrombosis: Dispelling myths. *Semin Vasc Surg* 2005;18:148–152.

31. Mundy LM, Leet TL, Darst K, Schnitzler MA, Dunagan WC. Early mobilization of patients hospitalized with community-acquired pneumonia. *Chest* 2003;124:883–889.

32. Tucker D, Molsberger SC, Clark A. Walking for wellness: A collaborative program to maintain mobility in hospitalized older adults. *Geriatr Nurs* 2004;25(4):242–245.

33. Brown CJ, Foley KT, Lowman JT, Roth DL, Allman RM. Impact of a hospital walking program on function and community mobility. *J Am Geriatr Soc* 2012;60(Suppl. 4):S5.

34. Munasinghe RL, Nagappan V, Siddique M. Urinary catheters: A one-point restraint? *Ann Intern Med* 2003;138(3):238.

35. Holroyd-Leduc JM, Sands LP, Counsell SR, et al. Risk factors for indwelling urinary catheterization among older hospitalized patients without a specific medical indication for catheterization. *J Patient Saf* 2005;1:201–207.

36. Fisher SR, Galloway RV, Kuo YF, et al. Pilot study examining the association between ambulatory activity and falls among hospitalized older adults. *Arch Phys Med Rehabil* 2011;92(12):2090–2092.

37. Bailey P, Thomsen GE, Spuhler VJ, et al. Early activity is feasible and safe in respiratory failure patients. *Crit Care Med* 2007;35:139–145.

38. vonRenteln-Kruse W, Krause T. Incidence of in-hospital falls in geriatric patients before and after the introduction of an interdisciplinary team-based fall-prevention intervention. *J Am Geriatr Soc* 2007;55:2068–2074.

39. Inouye SK, Bogardus ST, Baker DI, Leo-Summers L, Cooney LM. The Hospital Elder Life Program: A model of care to prevent functional decline in older hospitalized patients. *J Am Geriatr Soc* 2000;48:1697–1706.

CHAPTER 11

PRESSURE ULCERS: A PRIMER FOR THE HOSPITALIST

Aimée D. Garcia

PRESSURE ULCERS ARE PREVALENT, MORBID, AVOIDABLE, AND PUT HOSPITALS AT FINANCIAL RISK

Pressure ulcers are defined by the National Pressure Ulcer Advisory Panel (NPUAP) as "localized injury to the skin and /or underlying tissue usually over a bony prominence, as a result of pressure, or pressure in combination with shear and/or friction" [1]. A hospital-acquired pressure ulcer (HAPU) is defined as any pressure ulcer noted 24 or more hours after admission. Although it is commonly thought that pressure ulcers occur mostly in long-term care, the acute care hospital is also a setting for pressure ulcer development with incidence rates between 0.4% and 38%, and prevalence estimated at 15% [2, 3]. If a pressure ulcer develops during a hospital course, it can increase the patient's length of stay by fivefold, and increase the cost of the hospitalization by $2000–$11,000 [2]. Pressure ulcers that occur during a hospital stay can be precipitated by a variety of factors, such as the acute illness that caused admission, nutritional issues, or lack of focus on the skin. Traditionally, the care of the skin and monitoring of preventive measures has been the focus of nursing, but physicians are required and expected to be aware of all aspects of the patient. Because of the high cost associated with HAPUs, in October 2008, CMS changed their reimbursement framework for pressure ulcers. If a patient presents to a hospital with intact skin and develops a pressure ulcer during that hospitalization, the hospital will not be paid for the higher Medicare Severity Diagnosis Related Group (MS-DRG). Also, if a patient presents with a stage I or stage II pressure ulcer, and progresses to a higher stage (i.e., III or IV), the hospital will not be paid for the

Hospitalists' Guide to the Care of Older Patients, Edited by Brent C. Williams, Preeti N. Malani, and David H. Wesorick.

higher MS-DRG. If a pressure ulcer is present on admission, it will require physician documentation of that pressure ulcer for the hospital to receive the higher MS-DRG. This makes it critical that the clinician evaluate the patient's skin and appropriately document any evidence of pressure ulcers upon admission [4]. The populations at highest risk for pressure ulcers are spinal cord injury patients, frail elderly, hip fracture patients that are required to be immobilized in braces and traction, and critically ill patients.

The pathogenesis of pressure ulcers includes not only *pressure*, but *friction, shearing*, and *moisture*, all of which affect the skin's tensile strength and increase susceptibility for breakdown. Friction occurs when one surface is sliding across another surface with force. This can occur in patients who are dragged across sheets, agitated patients scooting themselves in the bed, or a patient pushing themselves up in bed with their heels. Shearing occurs when the skin is adhered to a surface, but the body is sliding in another direction. An example is a patient in which the head of the bed is elevated above 30° and the patient begins to slide down. The patient's skin might adhere to the bed, but the body is sliding down, thereby causing a shear effect on the blood vessels and tissues in the area. Moisture is essential to healthy skin, but an excess of moisture can lead to maceration of tissue. In addition, urine and stool are caustic to skin and will lead to incontinence-associated dermatitis if left against the skin too long. Skin that is macerated is more susceptible to shear and friction.

IDENTIFYING PATIENTS AT RISK FOR PRESSURE ULCER FORMATION OR PROGRESSION

The key to preventing pressure ulcers in the acute care setting is early identification of at-risk patients. Pressure ulcers will occur whenever there is compression of soft tissue between a bony prominence and an external surface for a prolonged period of time. A patient can go from having intact skin to a full thickness area of skin breakdown in a matter of hours if pressure is not relieved. The risk of pressure ulcer development begins when the patient enters the hospital, and often before. For example, if a patient has sustained a hip fracture, they may have been in a prone position on a hard surface for a number of hours prior to being found, or before emergency services arrive. The transportation to a hospital in an ambulance occurs by means of a stretcher that does not have a pressure redistribution surface on it. Once the patient arrives at the Emergency Center, they frequently spend many hours in that department, again on a stretcher with no

TABLE 11.1   Risk Factors for Pressure Ulcer Development

Intrinsic

Limited mobility: SCI, hip fracture, dementia, CVA, progressive neurological disorders

Poor nutrition: Anorexia, poor dentition, delirium, disease process, loss of smell, dietary restrictions

Medications: Sedatives, diuretics, chronic steroids

Poverty or lack of access to food

Depression

Comorbidities: Diabetes mellitus, congestive heart failure, renal failure, malignancies, chronic obstructive pulmonary disease

Aging skin

Tobacco use

Extrinsic

Pressure: Wheelchair, bed, geri chair, stretcher

Friction: Heels on bed, sliding across sheets, agitated patient

Shear: Sliding down in bed

Moisture: Bowel and bladder incontinence, sweating, skin folds

SCI, Spinal cord injury; CVA, cerebrovascular accident.

pressure redistribution, and without the ability to be turned and repositioned on a scheduled time frame. In addition, intrinsic risk factors may also have an effect on the patient's risk of skin breakdown, including poor nutrition, tobacco use, and comorbidities, that limit mobility such as osteoarthritis, or cardiac or lung disease.

Common risk factors for pressure ulcer development are listed in Table 11.1. A more standardized approach to risk assessment used at many hospitals is the use of risk scales. The most common scales used in the United States are the Braden scale and the Norton scale. Of the two, the Braden scale is more widely used and is the more validated. The Braden scale identifies 6 components, including *sensory perception*, *activity*, *mobility*, *nutrition*, *moisture*, and *friction/shear* (Fig. 11.1). The maximum score is 23, and patients with scores 18 or below are considered to be at risk. Hospitalists should be familiar with these six components to help identify patients at moderate or high risk for developing pressure ulcers, at admission and throughout their hospital stay.

The following two case scenarios highlight each aspect of pressure ulcer prevention and treatment.

BRADEN SCALE FOR PREDICTING PRESSURE SORE RISK

Patient's Name _____   Evaluator's Name _____   Date of Assessment _____

	1	2	3	4			
SENSORY PERCEPTION ability to respond meaningfully to pressure-related discomfort	**1. Completely Limited** Unresponsive (does not moan, flinch, or grasp) to painful stimuli, due to diminished level of con-sciousness or sedation. OR limited ability to feel pain over most of body.	**2. Very Limited** Responds only to painful stimuli. Cannot communicate discomfort except by moaning or restlessness OR has a sensory impairment which limits the ability to feel pain or discomfort over ½ of body.	**3. Slightly Limited** Responds to verbal com-mands, but cannot always communicate discomfort or the need to be turned. OR has some sensory impairment which limits ability to feel pain or discomfort in 1 or 2 extremities.	**4. No Impairment** Responds to verbal commands. Has no sensory deficit which would limit ability to feel or voice pain or discomfort.			
MOISTURE degree to which skin is exposed to moisture	**1. Constantly Moist** Skin is kept moist almost constantly by perspiration, urine, etc. Dampness is detected every time patient is moved or turned.	**2. Very Moist** Skin is often, but not always moist. Linen must be changed at least once a shift.	**3. Occasionally Moist:** Skin is occasionally moist, requiring an extra linen change approximately once a day.	**4. Rarely Moist** Skin is usually dry, linen only requires changing at routine intervals.			
ACTIVITY degree of physical activity	**1. Bedfast** Confined to bed.	**2. Chairfast** Ability to walk severely limited or non-existent. Cannot bear own weight and/or must be assisted into chair or wheelchair.	**3. Walks Occasionally** Walks occasionally during day, but for very short distances, with or without assistance. Spends majority of each shift in bed or chair	**4. Walks Frequently** Walks outside room at least twice a day and inside room at least once every two hours during waking hours			
MOBILITY ability to change and control body position	**1. Completely Immobile** Does not make even slight changes in body or extremity position without assistance	**2. Very Limited** Makes occasional slight changes in body or extremity position but unable to make frequent or significant changes independently.	**3. Slightly Limited** Makes frequent though slight changes in body or extremity position independently.	**4. No Limitation** Makes major and frequent changes in position without assistance.			
NUTRITION usual food intake pattern	**1. Very Poor** Never eats a complete meal. Rarely eats more than ⅓ of any food offered. Eats 2 servings or less of protein (meat or dairy products) per day. Takes fluids poorly. Does not take a liquid dietary supplement OR is NPO and/or maintained on clear liquids or IV's for more than 5 days.	**2. Probably Inadequate** Rarely eats a complete meal and generally eats only about ½ of any food offered. Protein intake includes only 3 servings of meat or dairy products per day. Occasionally will take a dietary supplement OR receives less than optimum amount of liquid diet or tube feeding	**3. Adequate** Eats over half of most meals. Eats a total of 4 servings of protein (meat, dairy products) per day. Occasionally will refuse a meal, but will usually take a supplement when offered OR is on a tube feeding or TPN regimen which probably meets most of nutritional needs	**4. Excellent** Eats most of every meal. Never refuses a meal. Usually eats a total of 4 or more servings of meat and dairy products. Occasionally eats between meals. Does not require supplementation.			
FRICTION & SHEAR	**1. Problem** Requires moderate to maximum assistance in moving. Complete lifting without sliding against sheets is impossible. Frequently slides down in bed or chair, requiring frequent repositioning with maximum assistance. Spasticity, contractures or agitation leads to almost constant friction	**2. Potential Problem** Moves feebly or requires minimum assistance. During a move skin probably slides to some extent against sheets, chair, restraints or other devices. Maintains relatively good position in chair or bed most of the time but occasionally slides down.	**3. No Apparent Problem** Moves freely in bed and in chair independently and has sufficient muscle strength to lift up completely during move. Maintains good position in bed or chair.				
				Total Score			

Figure 11.1   Braden Scale for Predicting Pressure Sore Risk.

CASE STUDY 11.1

Mrs. S is an 85-year-old female who is admitted to the hospital with pneumonia. She is otherwise healthy except for osteoporosis, osteoarthritis of her low back, and mild cognitive impairment. She has been living independently with daily visits from her daughter. She spends most of the day doing crafts, reading, and watching TV. Though not identified at admission, she frequently loses urine when she coughs or sneezes. On admission, she is in bed, and conversant though somewhat short of breath, and has some trouble following all the questions.

Clinical questions: Is this woman at risk of developing a pressure ulcer during her hospital stay? To what degree? What are her major risk factors?

Discussion: Although this patient is living independently and fairly functional at baseline, she has mild impairments in all six components of the Braden scale—compromised ability to communicate discomfort, spends most of her time sitting, limited movement due to her osteoarthritis, probable undernutrition, moist skin, and will experience sheer and friction forces from hospital "bed rest."

Her Braden score is 16–17, putting her at moderate risk of developing pressure ulcers during her hospital stay. Her Braden Score is calculated as: *Sensory perception*: 3—slightly impaired; *Moisture*: 3—occasionally moist; *Activity*: 3—walks occasionally; *Mobility*: 3—slightly limited; *Nutrition*: 2–3: probably inadequate to adequate; *Friction/Shear*: 2—potential problem.

CASE STUDY 11.2

Mr. W is an 80-year-old male who is admitted to the hospital following a hip fracture he suffered that morning. He was found by a family member after having lain on the floor for at least 4 hours. He has a history of moderate congestive heart failure from ischemic heart disease with an ejection fraction of 25–30%, and chronic kidney disease with a baseline creatinine of 1.8. In the Emergency Room, his creatinine was above baseline at 2.2, he had a few crackles in his lungs, and peripheral edema. He is admitted to your service for stabilization prior to surgery. Upon examination, the patient has an area of partial thickness skin breakdown on the sacral area with surrounding dark tissue.

Clinical questions: The presence of a pressure ulcer identifies this patient as high risk; what questions are most likely to identify risk factors for progression of this pressure ulcer or formation of others? What are the most important risk factors to address on admission?

Discussion: This patient's immobility puts him at high risk for pressure ulcer formation and he already has skin breakdown present on the sacral area. A few additional questions at admission to elucidate his *cognition, continence*, and *nutrition status* will likely identify further risk factors that could be addressed during his hospital stay. His immobile status will make toileting an issue, putting him at risk for moisture as a risk factor. He will be in traction, which will affect his activity and bed mobility significantly, and he will be at risk for friction and shear, which can significantly worsen the area of breakdown already present. Also, the pain medications he will be given will likely affect his sensory perception and may affect his cognition.

His Braden score is 13, calculated as: *Sensory Perception*: 3—slightly impaired; *Moisture*: 2—very moist; *Activity*: 1—bedfast; *Mobility*: 2—very limited; *Nutrition*: 3—probably adequate; *Friction/Shear*: 2—potential problem.

Hospitalists should promote the use of a formal risk assessment scale on any patient "flagged" by a nurse or physician as potentially at risk, and presentation of the score results (usually by nursing staff) on rounds. By doing so, physicians will learn to more readily recognize patients at risk for pressure ulcers, nurses will become comfortable with briefly and efficiently communicating pressure ulcer risk to physicians using a common language, and care planning to ameliorate or follow-up risk can be carried out at the bedside during routine work rounds.

PREVENTION STRATEGIES

Prevention strategies should be implemented for patients at *moderate* (1–2 risk factors or Braden scale 14–18), or *high risk* (3+ risk factors or Braden scale <14). Basic prevention strategies should be used on all patients at moderate or high risk, and additional interventions are indicated for high-risk patients. Templates for orders that can be used on admission for patients at risk are included in Table 11.2. Orders should include attention to six areas: *Turning*, *Nutrition*, *Pressure off-loading*, *Mobilization*, *Moisture minimization*, and *Bed and chair surfaces*. Examples of orders following this six-component template for the two cases above are listed in Table 11.3.

Once at-risk patients have been identified, it is important to do a thorough assessment of the patient's skin. Identification of bony prominences and potential sites of skin breakdown are useful in targeting therapy. Offloading the patient does not require expensive equipment. The use of pillows can be very effective. Sites such as the heels, between the knees, and behind the back to keep patient on their side all alleviate pressure and prevent skin breakdown. A turning and repositioning schedule is also important for offloading. Although there are studies underway examining the effectiveness of different time schedules of turning, at the present, the standard of care is considered every 2 hours. The facility should have a policy on how the turning schedule will be implemented and monitored.

Nutrition is an important factor in prevention of skin breakdown. Many geriatric patients are nutritionally compromised. This may be secondary to poor dentition, lack of money, lack of access, medications, or medical

TABLE 11.2   Strategies for Prevention

All patients at moderate or high risk (1+ risk factors or Braden Scale <19):
- Turning and repositioning every 2 hours
- Addressing nutrition early
- Monitoring skin every shift
- Moisture barrier cream if patient is incontinent (petrolatum, zinc paste, commercial moisture barrier creams)
- Floating heels (pillows, heel protectors)
- Padding bony prominences
- Monitoring skin every shift

Patients at high risk (3+ risk factors or Braden scale <15)—All of the above listed strategies, plus:
- Pressure redistribution surface
  1. Patient with no skin breakdown, but high risk for skin breakdown
     ○ Level 1: Static air, gel, foam mattress or overlay
  2. Patient with multiple stage II's or large stage III on trunk
     ○ Level 2: Low air loss mattress or alternating pressure mattress
  3. Patient with no turning surfaces or post-flap patient
     ○ Level 3: High air loss mattress
- Pressure redistribution cushion for wheelchair/Gerichair/bedside chair

conditions that decrease appetite. If a patient is not able to give a history, family or caregivers might provide insight into the patient's nutritional intake and if there has been any weight loss. A baseline weight should be obtained upon admission and can be used as a marker for comparison if the patient's usual weight is known. Unfortunately, at this time, there is no biochemical marker that accurately identifies nutritional status. Serum albumin and prealbumin have traditionally been used as markers of nutritional status, but neither one accurately predict visceral protein stores. Serum albumin has a half-life of 12–21 days, and is affected by various conditions, including fluid status, stress, inflammation, and underlying medical conditions, making it a poor marker of visceral protein status. The prealbumin has a half-life of 2–3 days and is as also affected by inflammation or underlying medical conditions. Prealbumin levels can actually be maintained in the presence of malnutrition [5]. If nutritional compromise is identified through clinical evaluation, a nutrition consult should be obtained. The registered dietician can complete a nutritional assessment on the patient and put strategies in place to maximize nutrition. This is especially important if the patient already has a pressure ulcer, as the protein and fluid requirements increase in response to skin breakdown.

TABLE 11.3   Sample Admission Orders Specific to Pressure Ulcer Prevention

Moderate risk patients (Braden score of 14–18): Mrs. S

- *Turning* and repositioning every 2 hours
- *Nutrition consult* to assess her nutritional state and maximize her nutrition
- *Pressure off-loading*: Pillows under her legs supporting her knees to float her heels off the bed
  - *Mobilization*: Getting her up as soon as she is able
  - *Moisture*: Nursing staff to help toilet her to minimize her risk of moisture on skin
- *Bed/chair*: In addition, her bed was placed in a low position, and all medications were reviewed to minimize the risk of delirium and falls.

Improving patient mobility as soon as she is able will help to prevent skin breakdown and decrease the amount of deconditioning.

Early assessment of nutrition and interventions to maximize the nutrition of the patient is an important part of patient care

High-risk patients (Braden score <14): Mr. W

- *Turning* and repositioning every 2 hours
- *Nutrition consult* to assess his nutritional state and maximize his nutrition
- *Pressure off-loading*
  Pillows under his legs supporting his knees to float his heels off of the bed.
  Heel protectors to both heels.
- *Moisture/mobilization*: *Getting him up* as soon as he is able decrease soiling and improve his mobility.
- *Bed/chair surfaces*
  Level 1 pressure reduction surface, which in his case was a static air mattress overlay.
  Air cushion for his wheelchair and bedside chair once he is able to get into a chair.

In patients with hip fractures, a combination of heel protectors and offloading with pillows can be especially helpful since this population is at very high risk of developing heel ulcers.

Because of the partial thickness skin breakdown on the sacral area, this patient qualifies for a level 1 mattress, which would include a static air, viscoelastic foam mattress, or a gel mattress (examples include: memory foam and ROHO® mattress)

Once the patient transitions to the bedside chair after surgery, use of a foam, gel, or static air cushion will also be needed to protect the ischial tuberosities.

For immobilized patients, improving mobility as early in the hospital-ization as possible will have multiple benefits. Patients who remain in bed are at increased risk of deconditioning, infections, and skin breakdown. Physical therapy assessments and bedside treatments can be started until the patient is able to be transferred to another care setting where more intensive rehabili-tation can occur. It is important to remember that pressure redistribution cushions need to be provided for the wheelchair and bedside chair if the patient is not able to reposition themselves. Repositioning in a wheelchair must be done every hour as opposed to every 2 hours in the bed since the pressure is more focused on the ischial tuberosities in a seated position. The choice of which support surface to use for the bed and wheelchair can best be done with the guidance of a wound care specialist; hospitalists should be familiar with reimbursement guidelines from the Centers for Medicaid and Medicare Services (CMS) (Box 11.1) to ensure reimbursement is available for specialized surfaces. Finally, prevention involves maximization of the patient's underlying medical conditions. Conditions such as uncontrolled hypertension, diabetes, congestive heart failure, systemic infections and renal failure place a physiological stress on the body, and can put the patient in a state of catabolism. The more conditions affecting the individual, the more stress on the body, and that paired with the lower physiological reserves of an elderly patient makes that individual more susceptible to skin breakdown.

STAGING PRESSURE ULCERS

Staging of pressure ulcers can serve numerous functions. It is an important part of communication within the healthcare team, it documents the progress or worsening of a pressure ulcer, and determines reimbursement for treatment modalities and hospital DRGs. The physician has an independent duty to assess the patient's skin and determine the stage of the wound. The physician must also order appropriate therapeutic interventions based on each stage of pressure ulcer. Appropriate staging and documentation will provide better patient care, facilitate reimbursement, and help decrease litigation.

The National Pressure Ulcer Advisory Panel (NPUAP) definitions of pressure ulcer staging will be outlined in this section. Pressure ulcers at each stage are illustrated in Figure 11.2, along with basic elements of treatment.

Stage I

"Intact skin with nonblanchable redness of a localized area usually over a bony prominence." The key to this definition is that the skin is intact. If there is any break in the surface of the skin, it is no longer a stage I. Special attention must be paid to individuals with dark skin. A physical exam of high-risk patients must include a tactile assessment of the skin. In darker-pigmented patients, the presence of nonblanchable erythema may not be as prominent, but the patient may have skin areas that are warmer, cooler, tender, firm, or boggy indicating an area of stage I damage.

BOX *11.1*

SUPPORT SURFACE INDICATIONS AND CATEGORIES

Group 1: Mattresses and overlays. Support surfaces designed to either replace a standard hospital or home mattress or as an overlay placed on top of a standard hospital or home mattress. Products in this category include mattresses, pressure pads, and mattress overlays (foam, air, water, or gel).

Reimbursement: A group 1 support surface is covered if the patient is completely immobile. Otherwise, he or she must be partially immobile, or have any stage pressure ulcer and demonstrate one of the following conditions: impaired nutritional status, incontinence, altered sensory perception, or compromised circulatory status. A physician order must be obtained prior to delivery of the equipment and should be kept on file by the supplier.

Group 2: Enhanced mattresses. Support surfaces designed to either replace a standard hospital or home mattress or as an overlay on top of a standard hospital or home mattress. Products in this category include powered air flotation beds, powered pressure-reducing air mattresses, and nonpowered advanced pressure-reducing mattresses.

Reimbursement: A group 2 support surface is covered if the patient has a stage II pressure sore located on the trunk or pelvis, has been on a comprehensive pressure sore treatment program (which has included the use of an appropriate group 1 support surface for at least one month), and has sores that have worsened or remained the same over the past month. A group 2 support surface is also covered if the patient has large or multiple stage III or IV pressure sores on the trunk or pelvis, or if he or she has had a recent myocutaneous flap or skin graft for a pressure sore on the trunk or pelvis and has been on a group 2 or 3 support surface.

Group 3: Complete bed systems. Support surfaces are complete bed systems, known as air-fluidized beds, which use the circulation of filtered air through silicone beads.

Reimbursement: A group 3 support surface is covered if the patient has a stage III or stage IV pressure ulcer, is bedridden or chair-bound, would be institutionalized without the use of the group 3 support surface, the patient is under the close supervision of the patient's treating physician, at least 1 month of conservative treatment has been administered (including the use of a group 2 support surface), and a caregiver is available and willing to assist with patient care.

Source: https://www.cms.gov/ContractorLearningResources/downloads/JA1014.pdf.

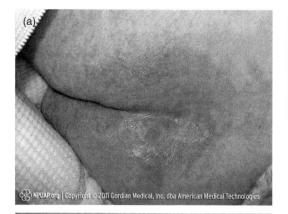

Treatment:

·turn and reposition every 2 hours

·moisture barrier cream *or* protective dressing, such as a hydrocolloid

·nursing to assess skin every shift

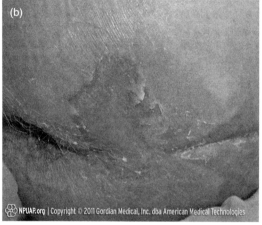

Treatment:

·turn and reposition every 2 hours

·moisture barrier cream *or* protective dressing such as a hydrocolloid or foam, if significant drainage (see table on dressings and indications)

·nursing to assess skin every shift

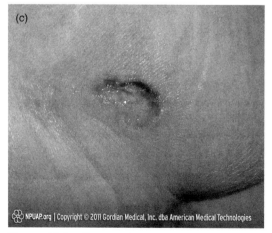

Treatment:

·turn and reposition every 2 hours

·moisture barrier cream to periwound

·dressing choice to wound based on tissue type and level of drainage (see table on dressings and indications)

·nursing to assess skin every shift

·assessment and maximization of nutrition

·level 1 matress (gel, foam, or static air overlay)

Figure 11.2   Stages of pressure ulcers and treatment plans. (a) Stage I: Nonblanchable erythema of intact skin. (b) Stage II: Partial thickness skin loss, no necrotic slough. (c) Stage III: Full thickness skin loss to the fascia, but not through the fascia. (d) Stage IV: Full thickness ulcer involving muscle, bone, or tendon. (e) Unstageable pressure ulcer. (f) Suspected deep tissue injury. (See color insert.)

191

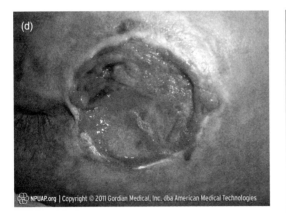

Treatment:

•turn and reposition every 2 hours

•moisture barrier cream to periwound

•dressing choice based on tissue type and level of drainage (see table on dressings and indications)

•nursing to assess skin every shift

•assessment and maximization of nutrition

•level 2 or 3 mattress (low air loss, alternating pressure, or high air loss); start with low air loss

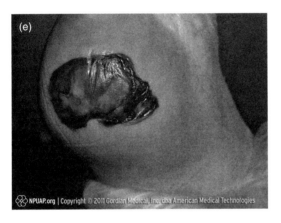

Treatment:

•turn and reposition every 2 hours

•dressing choice based on tissue type and level of drainage (see table on dressings and indications)

•nursing to assess skin every shift

•assessment and maximization of nutrition

•level 2 or 3 mattress if wound on trunk (low air loss, alternating pressure, or high air loss); start with low air loss

•debridement if slough or necrotic tissue is present

Figure 11.2 (*Continued*)

Stage II

"Partial thickness loss of dermis presenting as a shallow open ulcer with a red pink wound bed, without slough. May also present as an intact or open/ruptured serum-filled blister." A stage II is very superficial, and the wound bed is clean. There is no necrotic tissue within the wound bed. If a blister is present, it is filled with clear fluid. If the blister is filled with blood, it is not a stage II. A wound is also not identified as a stage II if the site is a skin tear, tape burn, perineal dermatitis, maceration, or excoriation (Fig. 11.2b).

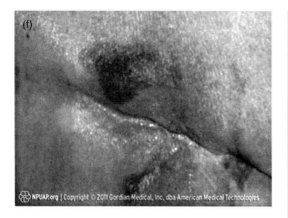

Treatment:

•turn and reposition every 2 hours

•when the skin begins to open, dressing choice based on tissue type and level of drainage (see table on dressings and indications)

•nursing to assess skin every shift

•assessment and maximization of nutrition

•because there is no break in skin, patient will not qualify for a specialty mattress under CMS guidelines. If the hospital owns its own pressure redistribution surfaces, the patient should be placed on it

•when the skin begins to open, debridement of necrotic tissue

Figure 11.2 (*Continued*)

Stage III

"Full thickness tissue loss. Subcutaneous fat may be visible but bone, tendon, or muscle is not exposed. Slough may be present but does not obscure the depth of tissue loss. May include undermining and tunneling." The depth of a stage III pressure ulcer will vary by the anatomical location. On the nose or ankle where there is very little subcutaneous tissue, a stage III may be very shallow. In an area such as the buttocks, a stage III may be very deep but still be in the subcutaneous tissue (Fig. 11.2c).

Stage IV

"Full thickness tissue loss with exposed bone, tendon, or muscle. Slough or eschar may be present on some parts of the wound bed. Often includes tunneling and undermining."

Deep Tissue Injury

"Purple or maroon localized area of discolored intact skin or blood-filled blister due to damage of underlying soft tissue from pressure and/or shear" (Fig. 11.2f).

Unstageable

"Full thickness tissue loss in which the base of the ulcer is covered by slough (yellow, tan, gray, green, or brown) and/or eschar (tan, brown, or black) in the wound bed."

If bone or tendon is exposed in a pressure ulcer, the clinician needs to maintain a moist wound environment to prevent the desiccation of those structures. Prompt surgical and wound care consultations for debridement of the wound bed and evaluation for treatment strategies are recommended.

An important aspect of staging is that wounds cannot be backstaged. If a wound is found to be at the subcutaneous level or deeper into muscle or bone, that wound is going to fill in with scar tissue. It is not the same structural integrity as a wound that is simply partial thickness and heals by reepithelialization. Appropriate documentation of a wound that begins as a stage IV, for example, but is now partial thickness would be to describe it as a "healing stage IV." Further description would state the tissue level at which it now presents. Underlying osteomyelitis needs to be considered whenever there is exposed bone or when a wound fails to progress despite appropriate interventions. This incidence of osteomyelitis when bone is probed is greater than 89%. It is appropriate to begin with a plain film of the affected area, but radiographic changes may not be evident for 2–4 weeks after onset of infection. Further workup will therefore be needed. A bone biopsy is ideal to evaluate the invading organism and target antibiotic therapy if the physician is able to obtain a specimen, but if there is not a physician able to do a bone biopsy, the next step is to obtain an MRI [6, 7].

DOCUMENTATION

Correct and thorough documentation of the wound is important when a patient has a pressure ulcer, not only for communication, but for reimbursement issues and litigation. The primary step is to determine if the ulcer that is present is truly a pressure ulcer. Conditions, such as skin tears, are not a result of pressure and should not be classified as a pressure ulcer. Incontinence-associated dermatitis or severe diarrhea, which can cause redness and superficial desquamation, can mistakenly be documented as a pressure ulcer. An abscess that has opened spontaneously can leave a defect resembling a pressure ulcer, but the clinical history will clarify the issue. It is better to describe a wound's appearance than to label it as a pressure ulcer if you are unsure.

Once a pressure ulcer has been identified, the clinician should provide a systematic, standardized documentation of the pressure ulcer, including six dimensions—*location, size, appearance of wound and periwound areas, type and amount of drainage, presence of odor, and tunneling or undermining*

TABLE 11.4   Documentation of a Wound

First, make sure it is a pressure ulcer . . .
Elements to be included in documentation of a wound:
- Location
- Size measured as length × width × depth in centimeters
- Appearance of wound bed
- Appearance of periwound
- Type of drainage
- Amount of drainage
- Presence or absence of odor
- Tunneling or undermining

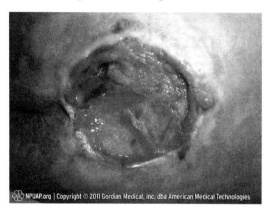

NPUAP.org | Copyright © 2011 Gordian Medical, Inc, dba American Medical Technologies

In this photograph, documentation of this wound would be:
15 cm × 18 cm × 1.0 cm at deepest point
100% pink/red tissue, no necrotic tissue, no slough
Periwound is intact and viable
Light serous drainage, no odor
Tunneling to 4 cm at 6:00

(Table 11.4). It is also important to reassess the patient on the same side each time, as the measurements of the wound can vary depending on positioning. Measurement of the wound can be challenging, as there is often variation between clinical staff. The standard measurement system goes on the premise that the wound is rectangular in shape [8]. The length is measured from the patient's head to foot at the longest point. The width is measured perpendicular to the length from side to side. The width is measured from the deepest point in the wound to the skin edge. All measurements are in centimeters. Depending on the capabilities of the facility, measurement techniques now include tracings and photographic assessments. The description of the wound bed itself is best accomplished by use of the red/yellow/black system. Red is the healthy, beefy red granulation tissue present in the wound bed. Yellow is slough or exudates that will require debridement. Black describes necrotic eschar. The tissue in the wound bed may not always be within this description parameter. If the wound tissue appears green, for example, due to bacterial colonization, accurate description on the wound bed would be to describe exactly what is noted. Each of the tissue types should be represented by a percent as seen by the examining clinician (e.g., 40% red, 30% yellow, 30% black). The periwound description can be categorized into viable, macerated, hyperkeratotic or necrotic tissue. For wound healing to progress, the periwound needs to have viable tissue present. Determination of the type and amount of wound drainage will require coordination with the nursing staff. The type of drainage can be described as serous, serosanguinous, sanguinous, or purulent. If the drainage changes from serous to another type, it might be an indication of erosion into deeper tissues, or of infection.

Documentation on the actual dressing of the date and time of the dressing change will help guide the clinician on the amount of drainage the wound is exuding. This will determine what type of dressing needs to be used to promote wound healing. If a wound is draining enough fluid that dressing changes three times a day are required, a highly absorbent dressing will be needed to promote moisture balance. The presence or absence of odor is frequently used as a marker of infection. Although odor might indicate a high bacterial load in the wound bed, many occlusive dressings, as well as dressings that had drainage, will have an odor. The odor in the wound bed cannot be determined until the dressing has been removed and the wound is thoroughly cleansed. Finally, a determination of tunneling and undermining needs to be done. Tunneling can be described as erosion into deeper tissues in which the base of the tract cannot be visualized, or from one structure to another. Undermining is destruction of tissue underneath intact skin, and often occurs at the edges of the wound [9]. Although tunneling can be described as depth in centimeters, tunneling is best described as the face of a clock. With the patient's head being 12:00 and feet being 6:00, the clinician should go around the edges of the wound documenting centimeters of defect. An example of documentation would be 3 cm of undermining at 5:00. Both tunneling and undermining are important in treating the wound as these areas need to be gently packed. If the superficial skin closes without the tunneling or undermining resolving, the site can become a potential source of an abscess formation. A documentation format has been outlined in Table 11.4.

All of the elements of a wound care assessment should be completed at the time that the pressure ulcer is documented and every week thereafter. The nursing staff should be monitoring the wound at dressing changes and during routine care, such as bathing and incontinence care. There should be communication with the attending physician if the wound characteristics change so that proper assessment can be achieved. It is not optimal for every member of the healthcare team to remove the dressing on daily rounds after a treatment plan has been initiated unless the nursing staff reports a change in wound status. Removal of the dressing exposes the wound to bacteria in the environment, and cools the surface of the wound, thereby impeding wound healing. Also, certain treatment modalities, such as enzymatic debridement, take time to work, so a clinician cannot expect a dramatic change in the wound bed in a few days.

A full assessment note of Mr. W's (Case Study 11.2) wound might look like:

5 cm × 4 cm × 0.1 cm stage II to sacrum

100% red tissue in wound bed. No surrounding erythema, periwound intact and viable. Minimal serous drainage, no odor. No evidence of tunneling or undermining.

PRESSURE ULCER TREATMENT: WOUND BED PREPARATION

In addition to contextual treatments (i.e., related to off-loading pressure, friction, moisture reducing, mobilization, and securing the most appropriate bed/chair surface), appropriate treatment for the wound itself—termed wound bed preparation—is critical. While specific therapies are often the purview of nurses or wound care specialists, hospitalists should be familiar with the basic elements of wound bed preparation to facilitate writing orders and communicating with other healthcare providers about pressure ulcer therapy.

There are four basic elements to wound bed preparation based on the TIME® principle of wound healing. These are tissue/debridement, infection/inflammation, moisture balance, and edge of wound [10].

Tissue Debridement

If necrotic tissue such as slough or eschar is present in the wound bed, it must be removed. Necrotic tissue increases inflammation, is a harbinger for bacteria, and delays wound healing. The level of necrotic tissue and the clinician's level of comfort will guide the treatment strategy. The most common forms of debridement are as follows:

- *Sharp debridement.* An instrument, such as a scalpel, scissors or dermal curette, is used to remove necrotic tissue from the wound bed.

- *Enzymatic debridement.* Use of an enzyme, such as collagenase, to enzymatically break down the necrotic tissue in the wound.
- *Biological debridement: use of larvae therapy.* Maggots are very effective in consuming only necrotic tissue, but their use is limited by access, as well as patient and clinician discomfort.
- *Autolytic debridement.* Use of an occlusive dressing or moist therapy in the wound bed to allow the body's own proteolytic enzymes to break down necrotic tissue. For autolytic debridement to be effective, moisture must be maintained in the wound bed.
- *Mechanical debridement.* Use of pulsatile lavage, whirlpool or wet-to-dry dressings to remove necrotic tissue from the wound.

Although the use of wet-to-dry dressings is a common practice, there has been extensive documentation in the literature that this form of debridement is not optimal. In long-term care facilities, surveyors will site the facility for suboptimal wound care if wet-to-dry is being ordered. It is strongly advised that wet-to-dry not be used as a form of mechanical debridement. Although gauze is inexpensive, nursing time is not, and a proper wet-to-dry dressing works on the premise that the dressing will dry in the wound bed, will be removed once the necrotic tissue is adhered to the dressing, and will be mechanically removed from the wound bed. This process has many inherent flaws. First of all, most wounds have an exudate, therefore, the dressing never truly dries. By maintaining moisture in the wound, the dressing is actually acting as an autolytic dressing. Second, a true wet-to-dry is going to require a three times a day dressing change, which is very labor intensive for nurses, and therefore very costly. In addition, because the tissue is being mechanically removed from the wound, it can be very painful for patients. Wet-to-dry is also not a selective form of debridement. Healthy granulation tissue can be removed along with the necrotic tissue [11].

So what type of debridement is ideal? In an acute care setting, sharp debridement is going to be the fastest and most effective form of debridement. A surgical consult will likely be necessary if the wound is large, requires OR debridement, or if there is concern about involvement of deeper structures. Superficial wounds with small amounts of necrotic tissue can be treated with enzymatic or autolytic debridement, with the understanding that these types of debridement are slower, but more selective.

Infection/Inflammation

If a wound has necrotic tissue or has been open for more than a few weeks, the likelihood that there is inflammation and/or infection in the wound impeding wound healing is high. Analysis of chronic wounds has demonstrated high levels of matrix metalloproteases (MMPs) and inflammatory mediators, which continuously degrade the basement membrane, maintain a high inflammatory state, and do not allow the wound to progress through the normal healing cascade. Often, removal of necrotic tissue, treatment to decrease bacterial load, or use of collagen dressings that bind MMPs will place the wound back into normal physiological balance and allow the wound to heal. In terms of infection, all wounds are colonized, but not all wounds are infected. If a wound shows poor healing, but there are no overt signs of systemic infection, it is likely to be critical colonization, meaning 1×10^5 bacteria are present in the wound bed and are negatively impacting wound healing. This type of colonization does not require systemic antibiotic therapy. A topical antimicrobial can be used locally to decrease bacterial load. Many dressings now available are effective in decreasing bacterial load, including silver dressings and cadexomer iodine. Topical antibiotics, such as bacitracin or mupirocin, can lead to bacterial resistance if overused. The use of agents such as chlorpactin, Dakin's, or betadine are toxic to healthy granulation tissue. These agents can be used for a short period of time to rapidly decrease bacterial load, but should be changed within 1–2 weeks to another agent to prevent fibroblast toxicity. A course of systemic antibiotics should only be used if clinical signs of cellulitis or systemic infection are present. It is also important to remember that in the geriatric patient, the only signs of systemic infection may be a change in functional or mental status. Consultation with an infectious disease specialist may be appropriate if there is clinical suspicion that a wound infection requiring IV antibiotics is present.

Moisture Balance

Moisture is needed for wounds to progress to healing. The key is balance. Too much moisture leads to maceration of the tissue, and too little leads to desiccation. The clinician needs to choose their treatment plan based on the level of drainage. If the patient has a highly exudating wound, a dressing that is highly absorbent is going to be required. If a wound is dry, a dressing that lends moisture to the wound bed is necessary. A list of dressing categories and their indications has been provided in Table 11.5. The clinician should become familiar with the dressings available in their facility so they can order appropriate treatments for patient care.

Edge

Keratinocytes are cells that are critical to wound closure. These cells are found at the wound edge, therefore particular attention needs to be paid to

TABLE 11.5   Five Main Dressing Types and Indications

1. *Hydrogels.* Dressings that lend moisture to the wound bed. They can come in the form of an aqueous gel, a permeated gauze, or a sheet. This type of dressing is used for wounds that need moisture. They are very soothing and cool, so ideal for radiation burns, donor sites, or clean wounds with good granulation tissue that require a moist wound environment to promote healing.
   (a) Gel: Change BID.
   (b) Gauze: Change BID.
   (c) Sheet: Change every other day.
2. *Hydrocolloid-occlusive dressing.* It has a low moisture vapor permeability so only good for wounds with low exudate. Because it is occlusive, this type of dressing can be used for autolytic debridement. Cannot be used with a deep wound. It is very adherent, so frequent dressing changes can cause tearing of the skin. Should never be used for skin tears. It is thick and can be used over pressure sites to protect the area.
   Dressing: Various sizes and shapes; change every 3–7 days (ideally 5–7 days).
3. *Film-occlusive dressing.* It is the type of dressing you will see used over an IV site. It also has a low moisture vapor permeability, so it retains moisture against the wound bed. It is very adherent, so frequent dressing changes can cause tearing of the skin. Should never be used for skin tears. It is very thin. It can be used on the sacral area to prevent shearing effect.
   Dressing: Change every 3–7 days.
4. *Alginates.* Made from brown seaweed. This dressing is absorbent, so it is good for a wound that has drainage. As it absorbs drainage, it becomes a gel, thereby providing moisture balance to the wound bed. It has to be in contact with the wound. Because of the gel properties, it will help with autolytic debridement of slough in the wound.
   Dressing: Change every 2–3 days depending on drainage.
5. *Foam.* Absorbent dressings. This type of dressing comes in a variety of shapes and sizes and is appropriate for a light to moderately exudating wounds. There are varieties of foam dressings that are highly absorbent and can be used for highly exudating wounds.
   Dressing: Change every 3–7 days depending on drainage.

this area to ensure that a viable edge is present. Common problems noted with wound edges are maceration, hyperkeratinization, and necrosis. Maceration is going to be present if there is too much moisture in the wound. Proper management of fluid balance will prevent maceration of the wound edge. Hyperkeratinization or callous is present in weight-bearing areas and indicates too much pressure on the wound. This calloused area will require debridement to a healthy edge. This type of tissue tends to reform, so serial debridements will likely be necessary. A necrotic edge indicates further tissue death. Depending on the anatomic site, a vascular assessment needs to be done, and debridement of the nonviable tissue performed if adequate blood flow has been established. If the site is on a lower extremity, and there is significant arterial compromise, ongoing debridement is only going to create a larger wound that would not be able to heal due to lack of adequate perfusion.

GOALS OF TREATMENT/DISCHARGE STRATEGIES

When dealing with geriatric patients, it is always important to establish goals of treatment with the patient and/or the family. A plan of care may be very different if the goal of treatment is palliation versus aggressive debridement. It is important to understand the patient's underlying medical conditions and how this is affecting wound healing and the potential for further skin breakdown. The patient and family need to be involved in the discussion, and the clinician must have an understanding of what the family's expectations are. This should be documented in the patient's record. For a patient who is hospice or at the end of life, it may be appropriate to recommend that the patient be turned less frequently, and that dressing changes be minimized for patient comfort, especially if turning the patient or dressing changes are painful. There are charcoal-based dressings that can be used on top of the wound to minimize odor, and various antimicrobial dressings can be used to decrease bacterial load. Pain should be aggressively managed, and topical anesthetic agents can be put into the wound bed to decrease discomfort. Although nutrition is important for wound healing, fluids and supplements that might be given to a patient to help heal a wound might increase secretions and urination, thus causing patient discomfort. Nutrition should be tailored to the patient's ability to intake food and liquids, and to their wishes [12].

Once discharge of the patient is imminent, early consultation with the social worker or case manager will facilitate transition of care. It will be necessary to determine what type of care setting the patient will require. This will depend on their clinical status, level of social support, and their level of skilled need. The clinician will need to coordinate care with the next care team and outline an appropriate plan for pressure ulcer treatment. This includes obtaining a specialty support surface for home use if medically necessary, and ordering home health for continued care. If the patient will be going home, the clinician should consider coordination with an outpatient wound care center to monitor the progress of the patient's wound.

CONCLUSION

The aging population is going to bring more elderly patients into the acute hospital setting and into the care of busy hospitalists. Changes in reimbursement are requiring the physicians to be the primary documenter of the patient's skin exam. The focus of this chapter is to provide the hospitalists with the tools necessary to properly assess patient risk, put preventive strategies in place, and document any pressure ulcers in a concise and thorough manner. In the same manner that we consult experts in the field of cardiology or critical care, we should be looking to our colleagues who are specialists in the field of wound care to manage these complex wounds. However, hospitalists should be able to initiate care and make sure that all elements of comprehensive patient care have been addressed, and coordinate the care of the specialist in the treatment of pressure ulcers.

REFERENCES

1. National Pressure Ulcer Advisory Panel. Pressure ulcer stages revised by NPUAP. 2007. Available at: http://www.npuap.org/pr2.htm (accessed April 11, 2013).
2. National Pressure Ulcer Advisory Panel. *Pressure Ulcers in America: Prevalence, Incidence, and Implications for the Future*, Cuddigan J, Ayello E, Sussman C (eds.). Reston, VA: NPUAP, 2001.
3. Cuddigan J, Berlowitz D, Ayello E. Pressure ulcers in America: Prevalence, incidence, and implications for the future: An executive summary of the National Pressure Ulcer Advisory Panel monograph. *Adv Skin Wound Care* 2001;14:208–215.
4. Centers for Medicare and Medicaid. Changes to the Hospital Inpatient Prospective Payment Systems and Fiscal Year 2008 Rates. October 2, 2007. Available at: http://www. cms.hhs.gov/AcuteInpatientPPS/downloads/CMS-1533-FC.pdf; pp. 311–317 (accessed April 11, 2013).
5. Posthauer ME, Dorner B, Collins N. Nutrition: A critical component of wound healing. *Adv Skin Wound Care* 2010;23(12):560–572.
6. Kapoor A, Page S, LaValley M, et al. Magnetic resonance imaging for diagnosing foot osteomyelitis. *Arch Intern Med* 2007;167:125–132.
7. Sugarman B, Hawes S, Musher DM, et al. Osteomyelitis beneath pressure sores. *Arch Intern Med* 1983;143:683–688.
8. Goldman RJ, Salcido R. More than one way to measure a wound: An overview of tools and techniques. *Adv Skin Wound Care* 2002;15:236–243.
9. Hess CT. The art of wound care documentation. *Adv Skin Wound Care* 2005;18:43–53.
10. Schultz GS, Sibbald RG, Falanga V, et al. Wound bed preparation: A systematic approach to wound management. *Wound Repair Regen* 2003;11(Suppl. 1):S1–S28.
11. Ovington LG. Hanging wet-to-dry out to dry. *Home Healthc Nurse* 2001;19(8): 477–483.
12. Langemo DK. When the goal is palliative care. *Adv Skin Wound Care* 2006;19(148): 150–154.

CHAPTER 12

DELIRIUM

Tia R.M. Kostas
James L. Rudolph

INTRODUCTION

Delirium is an acute, fluctuating disturbance of consciousness and cognition [1]. Hospitalized patients frequently suffer from delirium, with typical occurrence rates in medical inpatients of 20–30% [2], postoperative patients up to approximately 50% [3], and elderly intensive care unit (ICU) patients 70% [4]. Delirious inpatients have increased mortality, risk of institutionalization [5], risk of postoperative complications [6], length of stay [7], length of intensive care unit stays [8], and rates of long-term functional and cognitive decline. As a result, delirium adds significant cost to hospitalizations and subsequent medical care [9]. The high morbidity and mortality associated with delirium makes early diagnosis of delirium critical. Healthcare workers frequently fail to recognize delirium [10]. Age over 80, dementia, severe illness, dehydration, and sensory impairment increase the risk of underrecognition of delirium [11, 12].

There are two variants of delirium: the hyperactive (agitated) variant, and the hypoactive (quiet) variant. The hyperactive variant, which accounts for only about 25% of cases, is rarely missed, because the patient disrupts the flow of care [13]. The more common hypoactive variant is often missed because the patient is neither disruptive nor threatening [11]. For example, a patient with hypoactive delirium might briefly waken when addressed and comply with some requests, but then quickly fall back to sleep. Several studies have found that the hypoactive variant is detected less frequently and carries a higher mortality, in part due to the delay in diagnosis [11, 14, 15].

Because of the high morbidity and mortality associated with delirium, optimal hospital practices should include a system to identify high-risk patients, prevent delirium, monitor for delirium, assess for and treat precipitants of delirium, and appropriately treat and manage associated agitation. Figure 12.1 illustrates a checklist for the hospitalist to help prevent, identify, and manage delirium.

Hospitalists' Guide to the Care of Older Patients, Edited by Brent C. Williams, Preeti N. Malani, and David H. Wesorick.

I.   Identify risk factors (all patients over age 65 on admission)
  ___ Mini-cog
  ___ Screen for vision/hearing impairment (ask patient/family)
  ___ ADLs/IADLs
  ___ Admission labs with significant abnormalities
II. Utilize Prevention Strategies (daily in all patients over age 65)
  ___ Frequent orientation, clock and calendar in room
  ___ Minimize nighttime vitals, medications, procedures
  ___ Glasses and hearing aids at bedside
  ___ Ambulation three times daily
  ___ D/c catheters, lines as soon as possible
  ___ Review medication list, minimize medications that precipitate delirium
  ___ Assess and treat constipation
  ___ Assess and treat pain
  ___ Assess and treat dehydration
III. Monitor for delirium (daily in patients with at least 1 risk factor)
  ___ Modified RASS (if score ≠ 0 or changes ≥ 1 point, apply CAM)
IV. Diagnose delirium
  ___ apply CAM to patients with abnormal modified RASS
V.   Treat delirium (patients with positive CAM)
  a.   Identify and treat cause of delirium (patients with positive CAM)
  ___ Interim history and physical examination
  ___ Review med list
  ___ Screen for electrolyte abnormalities
  ___ Rule out infection
  ___ Rule out urine/stool retention
  ___ Monitor for uncontrolled pain
  ___ Monitor for drug withdrawal
  ___ Rule out acute cardiac, respiratory, and neurological conditions
  b.   Nonpharmacologic
  ___ Enforce delirium prevention strategies above
  c.   Pharmacologic (only if nonpharmacologic fail)
  ___ Antipsychotics for acute agitation (haloperidol or atypical antipsychotics)
  ___ Benzodiazepines for acute agitation for alcohol withdrawal or
  contraindication to antipsychotics

Figure 12.1   Hospitalists' checklist to prevent, identify, and manage delirium. ADLs, activities of daily living; IADLs, instrumental activities of daily living; CAM, Confusion Assessment Method; RASS, Richmond Agitation and Sedation Scale.

ADMISSION ASSESSMENT: IDENTIFYING PATIENTS AT RISK FOR DELIRIUM

Hospitalists should recognize patients who are at increased risk for delirium. Table 12.1 summarizes the major risk factors for delirium, which are discussed in detail below.

TABLE 12.1   Risk Factors for Delirium

Risk factor	Odds ratio, 95% CI
Fracture on admission	6.57 (2.23, 19.34)
Cognitive impairment	6.30 (2.89, 13.74)
Age over 80	5.22 (2.61, 10.44)
Illness severity (APACHE)	3.49 (1.48, 8.23)
Age over 65	3.03 (1.19, 7.71)
Infection	2.96 (1.42, 6.16)
Visual impairment	1.70 (1.01, 2.85)

Adapted from *DELIRIUM: Diagnosis, Prevention and Management Clinical Guideline 103*, National Institute for Health and Clinical Excellence. 2010, National Clinical Guideline Center: Regent's Park, London. p. 244 [22].
APACHE, Acute Physiology and Chronic Health Evaluation.

Preexisting Cognitive Impairment

The most common independent risk factor for delirium across studies is preexisting cognitive impairment. Thus, a detailed history, including input from informed caregivers, along with standardized cognitive screening at hospital admission, is beneficial to establish a patient's cognitive baseline. We recommend that hospitalists do not rely solely on orientation items and observation of usual conversation to assess for baseline cognitive deficits. The Mini-Cog is a brief cognitive screen that is short, can be administered by hospitalists within the usual workflow, and tests attention, memory, and executive function [16]. We recommend hospitalists or other care providers perform the Mini-Cog on all patients >65 years old. Many other cognitive screening tests are available (see Chapter 3); however, we prefer the Mini-Cog for its brevity, high sensitivity, and lack of education or language bias [16].

Sensory Impairment

In many older patients, the five senses decline with age. The combination of decreased sensory input (e.g., no glasses or hearing aids), cognitive impairment, and the unfamiliar hospital environment may lead to misinterpretation of communication (i.e., talking back to the television), alarms (i.e., telephone ringing), and elements of the environment (i.e., window is a picture frame). Impairments in vision and hearing increase the risk of delirium in hospitalized patients [17]. As a result, admission assessment should include evaluation of vision and hearing by asking patients about deficits, encouraging the use of hearing aids and glasses if patients use them at home, and looking in the ears for cerumen impaction. Other members of the care team should be alerted if a patient has significant sensory deficits that may affect their care (e.g., significant hearing loss).

Low Functional Performance

A patient's functional status can be an important predictor of many things, including the need for home services, institutionalization, and even death. Preadmission functional status is an independent risk factor for delirium after noncardiac surgery [18]. The activities of daily living (ADLs) and the instrumental activities of daily living (IADLs) provide an understanding of baseline function. ADLs measure the ability to perform seven basic care skills (feeding, bathing, grooming, dressing, toileting, transferring, and walking) [19]. The IADLs assess the ability to perform seven complex activities (using the telephone, grocery shopping, using transportation, cooking, housekeeping, taking medications, and handling finances) [20]. In addition to providing risk stratification for delirium, assessing this historical baseline information can inform the patient, the family, and the medical team about the expected course of recovery.

Comorbidities

While preexisting cognitive impairment is the strongest risk factor for delirium, other types of insults to the brain also likely predispose to delirium. A preoperative prediction rule developed for delirium after cardiac surgery found that depression, prior stroke, or prior transient ischemic attack are also risk factors for delirium [21]. Additionally, prior alcohol abuse, even in the face of subsequent abstinence, has been independently associated with delirium [18].

Abnormal Laboratory Values

In a delirium prediction rule for medical patients, blood urea nitrogen to creatinine ratio ≥ 18, a marker of dehydration, is associated with incident delirium [17]. Severe illness evidenced by the Acute Physiology and Chronic Health Evaluation II (APACHE) score has been found to predict increased risk of delirium [17, 22]; the APACHE II risk prediction tool takes into account age, as well as key lab values such as arterial pH, serum sodium, potassium, creatinine, hematocrit, white blood cells, and PaO_2 [23]. These abnormal laboratory values may represent underlying severe disease, organ system dysfunction, and/or an underlying vulnerability to stressors.

PRECIPITATING FACTORS FOR DELIRIUM

Medications

During the course of a hospitalization, numerous medications with central nervous system side effects are often given to patients; many of these can precipitate delirium and are illustrated in Table 12.2. The addition of more than three new medications is associated with a nearly threefold increase in the risk of developing delirium [24].

Pain medications may precipitate delirium, particularly meperidine, which increases the odds of delirium relative to other opioids [25]. Oftentimes, opioid medications are necessary for pain control; however, the clinically important point is to recognize the risk for delirium associated with opioid medications, necessitating low starting doses and close monitoring, especially in older patients with baseline cognitive impairment.

While opioids may precipitate delirium, uncontrolled pain can also precipitate delirium [25]. When pain medication is required in cognitively impaired patients, strong consideration should be given to scheduled pain medication, since patients will often not ask for medications ordered as-needed (PRN); furthermore, administration on a schedule has been shown to reduce total dose needs relative to PRN dosing [26]. We recommend first initiating scheduled acetaminophen for pain control in older patients without a contraindication. Acetaminophen has been shown to reduce total opioid needs and improve patient reports of pain in a postoperative randomized controlled trial [27]. One advantage of acetaminophen is its limited cognitive side effects compared with opioids. However, opioid pain medication is often required in hospitalized elders. We recommend using a low, standing initial dose (oxycodone 2.5 mg Q6h) for opioid-naive older patients with pain. Patient-controlled analgesia can improve pain control; however, caution should be used in older patients with cognitive impairment and those who have developed delirium, since their ability to self-administer

TABLE 12.2 Medications That Can Precipitate Delirium

Benzodiazepines
Anticholinergic medications
Diphenhydramine and other antihistamines
MEperidine
Digoxin and other centrally acting cardiac medications
Steroids

medication is usually impaired [28]. In summary, sedative use should be minimized, and analgesia should be carefully administered to minimize systemic exposure to opioids with psychoactive properties while adequately controlling pain.

Benzodiazepines are associated with an increased risk of precipitating delirium. It is important to keep in mind, however, that benzodiazepine withdrawal in patients who take benzodiazepines chronically can precipitate delirium as well. In the ICU setting, sedatives such as benzodiazepines or propofol are often given. However, two recent studies have found that the use of dexmedetomidine, an alpha-2 adrenergic receptor agonist that is used for sedation in the ICU setting, has a reduced rate of delirium compared with midazolam and lorazepam [29, 30]. Thus, the use of dexmedetomidine over benzodiazepines for sedation in the ICU setting may reduce the risk of delirium [31]. Benzodiazepine and sedative use in hospitalized elders may be minimized by improving sleep hygiene using nonpharmacological measures, such as decreasing environmental noise, creating a relaxing environment with minimal interruptions, thus trying to preserve the circadian rhythm [32].

Medications with anticholinergic side effects are commonly used in the inpatient setting; confusion is a well-known anticholinergic side effect. Antihistamines, especially first-generation H1 antagonists, such as diphenhydramine, are extremely anticholinergic and thus are known for precipitating delirium. Second-generation H1 antagonists, such as loratidine, and H2 antagonists, such as ranitidine, can also have anticholinergic side effects but generally to a lesser extent. Other medications that have potent anticholinergic side effects include tricyclic antidepressants, such as amitriptyline and nortriptyline, and antispasmodics, such as oxybutynin and tolterodine. We recommend avoiding medications that are strongly anticholinergic whenever possible in geriatric populations.

Some cardiac medications also can be centrally acting and should be used with caution, especially in older adults. For instance, digoxin can cause hallucinations and confusion; older patients are at an increased risk of digoxin toxicity, especially in doses >0.125 mg a day, due to diminished renal clearance. Furthermore, inotropic agents, such as dopamine and norepinephrine, deliver supraphysiologic doses of neurotransmitters that may travel centrally and affect cognition, increasing the likelihood of paranoia and delirium.

Lastly, corticosteroids are associated with potential psychiatric side effects including depression, hypomania, and psychosis. Older patients who require treatment with corticosteroids, especially with high doses, should be monitored closely for the development of delirium or other psychiatric side effects.

Hospital Environment

The hospital environment can be very disorienting for patients. Aging is associated with notable changes in sleep, including earlier awakening, increased sleep fragmentation, and reduced total time asleep [33]. Preservation of the sleep–wake cycle (minimized nighttime interruptions, adequate lighting, and sleep hygiene) may minimize precipitation of delirium [32, 34]. Existing data suggests that sleep deprivation is a plausible precipitant of delirium [35]. Consideration should be given to balance the patient's monitoring needs with the sleep requirements of the patient (i.e., Does the patient need a standing order for vital signs at midnight and 4 a.m.?).

Patients requiring ICU care are exposed to an even more disruptive environment; it is busy, noisy, light filled, and patients are approached, assessed, and stimulated constantly. Recent work in the ICU setting found that the environment may contribute to delirium through sleep deprivation and overstimulation [36]. While this environment is often required for a period of time, early transfer to less intense wards should be considered whenever possible.

Iatrogenic Events

Complications of hospitalization and surgery can precipitate delirium. For example, a leading identifiable cause of delirium in older inpatients is urinary tract infection associated with catheter use [24]. The use of a bladder catheter nearly triples the risk of delirium [24]. The use of restraints confers a more than fourfold increased risk of delirium [24]. Furthermore, reduced mobility through formal restraints or informal tethers (i.e., intravenous lines, oxygen tubing, and urinary catheters) can contribute to loss of function, falls, and increased rehabilitation placement [37]. We recommend avoiding bladder catheters and restraints as much as possible (and discontinuing as soon as medically appropriate). Furthermore, hospitalists must be vigilant to avoid preventable medical processes, such as deep venous thrombosis, pressure ulcers, deconditioning, malnutrition, and dehydration using a team-based approach [34].

MITIGATING RISK FACTORS TO PREVENT DELIRIUM

Nonpharmacological Interventions

Delirium can be prevented in inpatients by targeting at-risk patients with nonpharmacological interventions to improve baseline vulnerabilities and avoid iatrogenic complications [32, 34]. Many of these interventions need to be systematic and involve the whole inpatient team, especially nursing staff; thus, staff education on delirium prevention is critical. Nurse-led multidisciplinary rounds have been shown to reduce unnecessary urinary catheter use [38], which is important in preventing and treating delirium. Standard protocols for managing cognitive impairment, sleep deprivation, immobility, visual impairment, hearing impairment, and dehydration have been shown to decrease the incidence of delirium, the total number of days with and episodes of delirium, and number of sleep medications used [32]. A summary of interventions for prevention of postoperative delirium based on successful prevention models is presented in Table 12.3.

Though delirium prevention necessitates a team-based approach, individual hospitalists also have an important role. For all inpatients 65 and older, hospitalists should verify at least daily that patients' pain, constipation, and fluid status are managed appropriately. Medications that can precipitate delirium should be avoided. Hospitalists should order the removal of catheters and lines and avoid the use of restraints as much as possible. Finally, hospitalists should ensure that they have ordered patients' medications and vital signs in a way that they are timed appropriately, and not in the middle of the night, if possible.

Patients that demonstrate risk factors for delirium on their admission screening should receive extra attention to prevent delirium. Ideally, hospital rooms and work flow should be organized to minimize interruptive noise, keep patients upright with unobstructed vision, and maximize functional lighting. Nursing staff should be educated to reorient patients and communicate the schedule on a daily basis, to encourage use of glasses and hearing aids, and to mobilize patients at least three times daily.

Pharmacological Prophylaxis

Pharmacological methods have not definitively been shown to prevent delirium. Some studies show that antipsychotics may have some benefit, but the data are still not clear. In a single-site study, prophylactic administration of haloperidol, a high-potency dopamine antagonist, did not reduce the incidence of delirium after hip fracture, but did decrease the severity and duration of delirium [39]. Another study in elderly patients undergoing joint-replacement surgery found that administration of perioperative olanzapine resulted in a lower incidence of delirium, but when delirium did occur, it lasted longer and was more severe [40]. Furthermore, a study comparing a high-potency antipsychotic, an atypical antipsychotic, and placebo in ICU patients found no difference in the days alive without delirium [41]. As a result of these and other studies, the practice of prophylaxis with

TABLE 12.3   Prevention and Nonpharmacological Treatment of Delirium in Hospitalized Patients [3, 32]

Module	Interventions
Cognitive stimulation	• Orientation (clock, calendar, orientation board) • Communicate day's schedule • Avoid cognitively active medications
Avoid sleep deprivation	• Relaxing nighttime environment, including warm drink, pleasant music, massage • Nighttime noise reduction (silent pill crushers, vibrating beepers) • Time medications, vital signs, procedures appropriately
Improve sensory input	• Glasses, magnifying glasses, large-print books, illuminated telephone keypads • Hearing aids/amplifiers, ear wax disimpaction
Mobilization	• Ambulation or active range-of-motion exercises three times daily • Minimize immobilizing equipment (restraints, bladder catheters)
Avoidance of psychoactive medication	• Elimination of unnecessary medications • Pain management protocol
Avoid dehydration	• Fluid management • Electrolyte monitoring and repletion • Early recognition of dehydration • Volume repletion • Adequate nutrition protocol
Avoidance of hospital complications	• Bowel protocol • Early removal of urinary catheters • Adequate central nervous system O2 delivery • Postoperative complication monitoring protocol

antipsychotics should be avoided due to increased risk of death, delirium, and other complications attributed to this class of drugs [42].

Acetylcholinesterase inhibitors are medications used to stabilize cognitive function in dementia. A randomized controlled trial of rivastigmine for delirium prevention in cardiac surgery found no effect of treatment on delirium incidence or cognitive performance [43]. In elective orthopedic surgery, the results have been mixed, with one trial showing no effect [44] and another suggesting benefit [45]. A randomized controlled trial of rivastigmine for delirium treatment was stopped early due to increased mortality in the treatment arm and no effect on delirium [46]. Thus, at this time, prevention or treatment of delirium with acetylcholinesterase inhibitors should be avoided as well [47].

MONITORING FOR DELIRIUM

Once admitted, patients with one or more risk factors should be monitored closely for delirium. A standardized strategy for monitoring patients for acute changes in attention, awareness, or activities should be considered. One group has proposed the creation of a mental status vital sign to identify changes rapidly [48]. A follow up study from this group found that longitudinal monitoring of consciousness using a modified version of the Richmond Agitation and Sedation Scale (RASS) can identify delirium (Fig. 12.2). Any score besides zero on the modified RASS is considered to be abnormal, and as a single assessment it has a sensitivity of 64% and a specificity of 93% for delirium [49]. However, the modified RASS is valuable as a monitoring

1. Administer Scale

State patient's name, ask patient to open eyes and look at speaker.
State, "Describe how you are feeling today."
If answer is short (<10s), cue with another open-ended question.
If no response to verbal cue, provide physical stimulation by shaking shoulder.

2. Score Scale

-5	**Unarousable** (no response to voice or physical stimulation)
-4	**Can't stay awake** (arousable but no attention; no response to voice but physical stimulation causes movement or eye opening)
-3	**Difficult to wake** (repeated calling/touch required for eye contact/attention, eye opening to voice but no eye contact)
-2	**Wakes slowly** (very drowsy, sometimes pays attention, briefly awakens with eye contact to voice <10s)
-1	**Wakes easily** (slightly drowsy, eye contact>10s, eye opening/contact to voice >10s, not fully alert but with sustained awakening,
0	**Alert and calm** (good attention and eye contact, responds immediately and appropriately to name/touch)
+1	**Restless** (slightly distractible, usually pays attention, anxious but cooperative)
+2	**Slightly agitated** (easily distractible, quickly loses attention, resists care/uncooperative, frequent non-purposeful movements)
+3	**Very agitated** (very distractible, aggressive, fights environment not people, repeated calling/touching required to maintain eye contact/attention)
+4	**Combative** (no attention, violent, danger to staff)

Figure 12.2   Modified Richmond Agitation and Sedation Scale. Any score besides 0 is abnormal. Adapted from Chester JG, Harrington MB, Rudolph JL. Serial administration of a modified Richmond Agitation and Sedation Scale for delirium screening. *J Hosp Med* 2012;7(5):450-453 [49].

tool over time to look for changes. When used to detect change, serial modified RASS assessments had a sensitivity of 74% and a specificity of 92% [49]. The key element is to have a rapid (<30 second) assessment of mental status in which changes are easily detected—similar to temperature or blood pressure. We advocate using a rapid assessment of cognition, such as the modified RASS on a daily basis in all patients over 65 with at least one risk factor for delirium. A score other than 0, or a change from the previous day's modified RASS score, would indicate a change in mental status and should be investigated.

DIAGNOSING DELIRIUM

Because of the morbidity associated with delirium, early identification of delirium is extremely important. A diagnostic algorithm, such as the criteria from the *Diagnostic and Statistical Manual of Mental Disorders, Fourth Edition, Text Revision* (DSM-IV-TR) or the Confusion Assessment Method (CAM), should be used. The DSM-IV-TR criteria include (a) disturbance of consciousness and attention, (b) change in cognition or the development of a perceptual disturbance, and (c) the disturbance is acute and fluctuating [1]. The CAM, which is based on DSM-IIIR criteria [50], has been demonstrated to be reliable, sensitive, and specific for diagnosing delirium compared with expert clinician examination [51, 52] after supplemental cognitive assessment. Please see Figure 12.3 for the CAM algorithm. We recommend using the CAM to identify delirium in patients who demonstrate abnormal modified RASS scores.

There are important elements of these tools that need to be clarified. Most importantly, attention is the core deficit in delirium, and must be carefully assessed when a diagnosis of delirium is entertained. Attention is best assessed when formal testing (digit span, months of the year backward, serial 7s, etc) is combined with interviewer observations instead of relying on either alone [53]. Notably, orientation items have low sensitivity for inattention and diagnosing delirium and should not be considered the standard assessment for attention [54].

The CAM-ICU is a delirium diagnostic tool that has been validated in nonverbal intensive care unit patients [55]. The CAM-ICU operationalizes the CAM by adding objective assessments for attention, consciousness, and thought [55]. The advantages of the CAM-ICU are that it can be performed by trained nurses or physicians; can be repeated over time to detect fluctuation and changes; and has been associated with ICU outcomes, including mortality [56], length of stay [57], and cost [58]. The key elements of the CAM-ICU are the Richmond Agitation and Sedation Scale, a validated

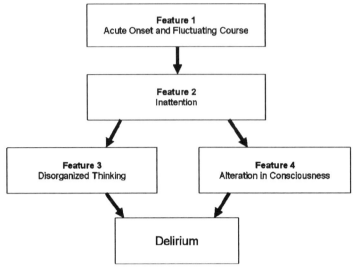

Figure 12.3   Delirium Algorithm-Confusion Assessment Method. The Confusion Assessment Method (CAM) algorithm. Patients are delirious when they have confusion along with Feature 1, Feature 2, and either Feature 3 or Feature 4 [51].

measure of consciousness [59], the Attention Screening Exam [60], and five thought questions.

Differentiating the Criteria for Delirium, Dementia, and Depression

In some cases, differentiating between delirium, depression, and dementia can be a challenge. Table 12.4 lists the clinical features that differentiate these three disorders. In the hospitalized setting, delirium should be assumed until proven otherwise. Dementia and depression cannot be diagnosed in the presence of delirium [1]. Thus, the historical understanding of prior cognition and functioning is important for the diagnosis of delirium. Cognitively, delirium can be distinguished from depression and dementia by the assessment of attention, which is generally preserved in mild and moderate depression and dementia.

TREATMENT OF DELIRIUM

Identify and Treat the Etiology

Given the high morbidity and mortality associated with delirium, delirium can be a medical emergency; thus, all patients with delirium should be

TABLE 12.4   Differentiating Delirium, Dementia, and Depression

	Delirium	Dementia	Depression
Onset	Acute	Chronic	Subacute/Chronic
Cognitive Domain(s)	Attention	Memory At least one of: Apraxia Aphasia Agnosia Executive dysfunction	Severe depression can cause variable deficits in cognitive function
Assessment	CAM, CAM-ICU, DSM-IV-TR criteria	MMSE, MoCA, neuropsychological testing	PHQ-9, GDS-15, Hospital Anxiety and Depression Scale (HADS) [75]
Diagnosis	CAM, DSM-IV-TR criteria	Neuropsychological testing, DSM-IV-TR criteria	DSM-IV-TR criteria
Morbidity	Institutionalization Decreased functional ability Prolonged cognitive sequelae Death	Institutionalization Decreased functional ability Death	Decreased functional ability [76]

CAM, Confusion Assessment Method; CAM-ICU, Confusion Assessment Method for the Intensive Care Unit; DSM-IV-TR, *Diagnostic and Statistical Manual of Mental Disorders; Fourth Edition, Text Revision*; MMSE, Mini Mental Status Exam; MoCA, Montreal Cognitive Assessment; PHQ-9, Nine-Item Depression Scale of the Patient Health Questionnaire; GDS-15, 15-item Geriatric Depression Scale; HADS, Hospital Anxiety and Depression Scale.

assessed promptly with an interim history, thorough physical exam with a focus on the neurological exam and looking for any potential sources of pain, and targeted laboratory testing based on the history and examination. Medications recently administered or withdrawn should be thoroughly reviewed. The initial aim in treating delirium is to identify and treat its underlying cause(s). Thus, the clinician should begin with a broad differential diagnosis and systematically eliminate potential causes. It is important to note that the causes of delirium are often multifactorial, and therefore the search for additional causes and contributors to delirium should not be terminated when a single cause has been identified (see Table 12.5).

Prior work has found that, in the absence of focal neurological deficits, a head CT has low diagnostic value in the assessment and treatment of the delirious patient [61]. MRI scanning is particularly difficult given the time and cooperation required. In the patient with delirium, sedation may be

TABLE 12.5   Differential Diagnosis of Delirium

Cause	Precipitating factors
Drugs	Anticholinergics
	Antihistamines
	Benzodiazepines
	Centrally acting cardiac medications
	Tricyclic antidepressants
	Dihydropyridines
	Inhaled anesthetics
	Meperidine
	Steroids
Electrolyte Abnormalities	Glucose
	Sodium
	Calcium
Lack of Sensory Input	Restraints
	ICU environment
	Hearing loss
	Vision loss
	Bed rest
Infection	Urinary tract infection (catheter-associated)
	Aspiration pneumonia
	Pressure ulcer
	Venous catheter infection
Retention (urine and fecal)	Medications
	Benign prostatic hypertrophy
	Severe constipation
	Dehydration
Intraoperative	Hypotension
	Embolization
	Delayed effects of anesthesia
	Medications
Under-dosing of drugs	Pain
	Alcohol withdrawal
	Withdrawal from chronic medications
	Gabapentin
	Antidepressants
	Benzodiazepines
Medical conditions	Myocardial infarction
	Pulmonary embolism
	Congestive heart failure
	Hypercarbia/hypoxia
	Uremia
	Acute stroke (usually other neurological signs present as well)

needed for imaging, which can worsen or prolong the delirium [62]. Thus, routine cerebral imaging is not recommended; imaging should be considered in those patients with new focal neurological findings or those at high risk of infarct or other intracranial pathology in whom no other cause can be identified.

Management of Agitation Associated with Delirium

When possible, management of delirium should begin by relieving the offending precipitant (constipation, urinary retention, etc.). Nonpharmacological interventions should also be initiated. For example, elimination of environmental noise, allowing the patient to sleep at night, and reorientation efforts should be implemented. A one-to-one "sitter" is always preferable to using restraints to ensure patient safety. Another useful resource is family, who can help provide reorientation and reassurance. Because of the low risk of adverse events, nonpharmacological methods are always recommended as a first step.

For patients in whom these nonpharmacological interventions are insufficient, antipsychotics are considered the first line for the pharmacological management of agitation associated with delirium [42, 63]. It is important to note that these medications do not treat delirium; they are simply helpful to manage the agitation associated with hyperactive delirium. For most patients, haloperidol at a low initial dosage of 0.5–1.0 mg orally is a reasonable choice. If there is no response within 1 hour, a repeat dosage may be considered. If there is no effect after 2–3 mg of haloperidol, it is unlikely that the patient is going to respond.

When administering antipsychotics, close attention must be paid to potential side effects. Antipsychotics administered in the acute setting have not been demonstrated to increase mortality, but even intermediate-term (6–12 weeks) use of antipsychotics are associated with increased mortality in some studies, especially among cognitively impaired patients [64, 65]. Additionally, electrocardiograms should be performed at baseline and used to monitor the QTc interval due to the risk of prolongation [66]. Finally, early evidence suggests that acute administration of antipsychotics may be associated with oropharyngeal dysphagia, which may further delay overall recovery [67]. At this time, there is no evidence for an incremental benefit of atypical antipsychotics beyond that of haloperidol for the treatment of delirium, though these are also reasonable options for delirium treatment [42].

For patients with contraindications to antipsychotics, such as Parkinson's disease, Lewy body dementia, prior seizures, and prior neuroleptic malignant syndrome, agitation may be managed with low-dose benzodiazepines. In general, benzodiazepines disinhibit patients; they should be monitored for a paradoxical reaction, in which administration of the benzo-diazepine results in agitation. Additionally, prior work has shown that benzodiazepines may actually prolong or worsen the course of delirium [62]. Finally, respiratory depression becomes a risk in older patients with respiratory comorbidities. Thus, other than the specific case of alcohol or chronic sedative withdrawal, use of benzodiazepines should not be considered a first-line therapy. If used, these agents should be reserved for cases where clinical circumstances limit use of antipsychotics.

IMPLICATIONS OF DELIRIUM BEYOND THE HOSPITAL STAY

While generally thought of as a short-term disorder, delirium can have lasting effects. First, delirium itself can persist for months. In a study of patients with delirium upon admission to a rehabilitation facility after hospitalization, delirium persisted for 6 months in one-third of patients [68]. Persistent delirium increased the 1-year mortality and prevented functional recovery [68, 69]. There is an increasing body of evidence that persistent delirium can delay both cognitive and functional recovery [5].

Delirium may have long-term mental health complications that are not fully studied and may impact functional recovery. Delirium may accelerate cognitive decline in patients with Alzheimer's disease [70]. Furthermore, evidence exists that patients who have an episode of delirium are at higher risk for the development of dementia [5]. In addition, newer evidence is emerging that younger patients with delirium may develop a posttraumatic stress disorder-like syndrome [71, 72]. Furthermore, sometimes patients who suffer from delirium during an acute hospitalization may have a preexisting dementia that was previously unrecognized. Thus, it is important that patients undergo formal cognitive assessment after the acute hospitalization and resolution of the delirium.

Lastly, delirium impacts the need for institutionalization. Patients who were not institutionalized prior to their episode of delirium are subsequently at higher risk for institutionalization [5]. Furthermore, several studies have demonstrated that postoperative delirium is associated with functional decline and nursing home placement 1–3 months after surgery [73, 74].

CONCLUSION

Delirium is an acute change in cognitive function, specifically attention, with associated disorganization of thought and abnormal level of consciousness.

Delirium is very common in hospitalized older patients and is associated with substantial morbidity, costs, and mortality. Admission delirium risk assessment is critical for the identification of patients who would most benefit from delirium prevention and surveillance protocols. Nonpharmacological delirium prevention strategies have proven effective at reducing delirium incidence, but pharmacological prevention strategies do not yet have trial-based support. The primary treatment of delirium is to identify and treat the underlying causes. Delirium has substantial long-term consequences, which are currently being better defined through large-scale epidemiological studies. Assessing delirium risk, employing delirium prevention strategies, and implementing standardized treatment protocols help provide optimal care for hospitalized older patients.

ACKNOWLEDGMENTS

Dr. Rudolph is supported by a VA Rehabilitation Research Career Development Award. Drs. Rudolph and Kostas are VA employees. Dr. Kostas has created and published an educational geriatric pocket card which she may receive royalties from in the future (none yet received). The authors have no other disclosures.

REFERENCES

1. *Diagnostic and Statistical Manual of Mental Disorders (DSM-IV-TR)*, 4th ed. Washington, DC: American Psychiatric Association, 2000.
2. Siddiqi N, House AO, Holmes JD. Occurrence and outcome of delirium in medical in-patients: A systematic literature review. *Age Ageing* 2006;35:350–364.
3. Rudolph JL, Marcantonio ER. Review articles: Postoperative delirium: Acute change with long-term implications. *Anesth Analg* 2011;112:1202–1211.
4. McNicoll L, Pisani MA, Zhang Y, Ely EW, Siegel MD, Inouye SK. Delirium in the intensive care unit: Occurrence and clinical course in older patients. *J Am Geriatr Soc* 2003;51:591–598.
5. Witlox J, Eurelings LS, de Jonghe JF, Kalisvaart KJ, Eikelenboom P, van Gool WA. Delirium in elderly patients and the risk of postdischarge mortality, institutionalization, and dementia: A meta-analysis. *JAMA* 2010;304:443–451.
6. Martin BJ, Buth KJ, Arora RC, Baskett RJ. Delirium as a predictor of sepsis in post-coronary artery bypass grafting patients: A retrospective cohort study. *Crit Care* 2010;14:R171.
7. Rudolph JL, Jones RN, Rasmussen LS, Silverstein JH, Inouye SK, Marcantonio ER. Independent vascular and cognitive risk factors for postoperative delirium. *Am J Med* 2007;120:807–813.
8. Norkiene I, Ringaitiene D, Misiuriene I, et al. Incidence and precipitating factors of delirium after coronary artery bypass grafting. *Scand Cardiovasc J* 2007;41:180–185.
9. Franco K, Litaker D, Locala J, Bronson D. The cost of delirium in the surgical patient. *Psychosomatics* 2001;42:68–73.

10. Gustafson Y, Brannstrom B, Norberg A, Bucht G, Winblad B. Underdiagnosis and poor documentation of acute confusional states in elderly hip fracture patients. *J Am Geriatr Soc* 1991;39:760–765.

11. Inouye SK, Foreman MD, Mion LC, Katz KH, Cooney LM, Jr. Nurses' recognition of delirium and its symptoms: Comparison of nurse and researcher ratings. *Arch Intern Med* 2001;161:2467–2473.

12. Rudolph JL, Harrington MB, Lucatorto MA, Chester JG, Francis J, Shay KJ. Validation of a medical record-based delirium risk assessment. *J Am Geriatr Soc* 2011;59: S289–S294.

13. Liptzin B, Levkoff SE. An empirical study of delirium subtypes. *Br J Psychiatry* 1992;161:843–845.

14. Levkoff SE, Evans DA, Liptzin B, et al. Delirium. The occurrence and persistence of symptoms among elderly hospitalized patients. *Arch Intern Med* 1992;152: 334–340.

15. Kiely DK, Jones RN, Bergmann MA, Marcantonio ER. Association between psychomotor activity delirium subtypes and mortality among newly admitted post-acute facility patients. *J Gerontol A Biol Sci Med Sci* 2007;62:174–179.

16. Borson S, Scanlan J, Brush M, Vitaliano P, Dokmak A. The mini-cog: A cognitive "vital signs" measure for dementia screening in multi-lingual elderly. *Int J Geriatr Psychiatry* 2000;15:1021–1027.

17. Inouye SK, Viscoli CM, Horwitz RI, Hurst LD, Tinetti ME. A predictive model for delirium in hospitalized elderly medical patients based on admission characteristics. *Ann Intern Med* 1993;119:474–481.

18. Marcantonio ER, Goldman L, Mangione CM, et al. A clinical prediction rule for delirium after elective noncardiac surgery. *JAMA* 1994;271:134–139.

19. Katz S, Downs TD, Cash HR, Grotz RC. Progress in development of the index of ADL. *Gerontologist* 1970;10:20–30.

20. Lawton MP, Brody EM. Assessment of older people: Self-maintaining and instrumental activities of daily living. *Gerontologist* 1969;9:179–186.

21. Rudolph JL, Jones RN, Levkoff SE, et al. Derivation and validation of a preoperative prediction rule for delirium after cardiac surgery. *Circulation* 2009;119:229–236.

22. DELIRIUM: diagnosis, prevention and management Clinical Guideline 103. National Institute for Health and Clinical Excellence. Regent's Park, London: National Clinical Guideline Centre; 2010. pp. 255–302.

23. Knaus WA, Draper EA, Wagner DP, Zimmerman JE. APACHE II: A severity of disease classification system. *Crit Care Med* 1985;13:818–829.

24. Inouye SK, Charpentier PA. Precipitating factors for delirium in hospitalized elderly persons. Predictive model and interrelationship with baseline vulnerability. *JAMA* 1996;275:852–857.

25. Marcantonio ER, Juarez G, Goldman L, et al. The relationship of postoperative delirium with psychoactive medications. *JAMA* 1994;272:1518–1522.

26. Paice JA, Noskin GA, Vanagunas A, Shott S. Efficacy and safety of scheduled dosing of opioid analgesics: A quality improvement study. *J Pain* 2005;6:639–643.

27. Schug SA, Sidebotham DA, McGuinnety M, Thomas J, Fox L. Acetaminophen as an adjunct to morphine by patient-controlled analgesia in the management of acute postoperative pain. *Anesth Analg* 1998;87:368–372.

28. Mann C, Pouzeratte Y, Boccara G, et al. Comparison of intravenous or epidural patient-controlled analgesia in the elderly after major abdominal surgery. *Anesthesiology* 2000;92:433–441.

29. Pandharipande PP, Pun BT, Herr DL, et al. Effect of sedation with dexmedetomidine vs lorazepam on acute brain dysfunction in mechanically ventilated patients: The MENDS randomized controlled trial. *JAMA* 2007;298:2644–2653.

30. Riker RR, Shehabi Y, Bokesch PM, et al. Dexmedetomidine vs midazolam for sedation of critically ill patients: A randomized trial. *JAMA* 2009;301:489–499.

31. Maldonado JR, Wysong A, van der Starre PJ, Block T, Miller C, Reitz BA. Dexmedetomidine and the reduction of postoperative delirium after cardiac surgery. *Psychosomatics* 2009;50:206–217.

32. Inouye SK, Bogardus ST, Jr., Charpentier PA, et al. A multicomponent intervention to prevent delirium in hospitalized older patients. *N Engl J Med* 1999;340:669–676.

33. Crowley K. Sleep and sleep disorders in older adults. *Neuropsychol Rev* 2011;21:41–53.

34. Marcantonio ER, Flacker JM, Wright RJ, Resnick NM. Reducing delirium after hip fracture: A randomized trial. *J Am Geriatr Soc* 2001;49:516–522.

35. Weinhouse GL, Schwab RJ, Watson PL, et al. Bench-to-bedside review: Delirium in ICU patients—Importance of sleep deprivation. *Crit Care* 2009;13:234.

36. Osse RJ, Tulen JH, Bogers AJ, Hengeveld MW. Disturbed circadian motor activity patterns in postcardiotomy delirium. *Psychiatry Clin Neurosci* 2009;63:56–64.

37. Inouye SK. Delirium in older persons. *N Engl J Med* 2006;354:1157–1165.

38. Fakih MG, Dueweke C, Meisner S, et al. Effect of nurse-led multidisciplinary rounds on reducing the unnecessary use of urinary catheterization in hospitalized patients. *Infect Control Hosp Epidemiol* 2008;29:815–819.

39. Kalisvaart KJ, de Jonghe JF, Bogaards MJ, et al. Haloperidol prophylaxis for elderly hip-surgery patients at risk for delirium: A randomized placebo-controlled study. *J Am Geriatr Soc* 2005;53:1658–1666.

40. Larsen KA, Kelly SE, Stern TA, et al. Administration of olanzapine to prevent postoperative delirium in elderly joint-replacement patients: A randomized, controlled trial. *Psychosomatics* 2010;51:409–418.

41. Girard TD, Pandharipande PP, Carson SS, et al. Feasibility, efficacy, and safety of antipsychotics for intensive care unit delirium: The MIND randomized, placebo-controlled trial. *Crit Care Med* 2010;38:428–437.

42. Lonergan E, Britton AM, Luxenberg J, Wyller T. Antipsychotics for delirium. *Cochrane Database Syst Rev* 2007;(2):CD005594.

43. Gamberini M, Bolliger D, Lurati Buse GA, et al. Rivastigmine for the prevention of postoperative delirium in elderly patients undergoing elective cardiac surgery—A randomized controlled trial. *Crit Care Med* 2009;37:1762–1768.

44. Liptzin B, Laki A, Garb JL, Fingeroth R, Krushell R. Donepezil in the prevention and treatment of post-surgical delirium. *Am J Geriatr Psychiatry* 2005;13:1100–1106.

45. Sampson EL, Raven PR, Ndhlovu PN, et al. A randomized, double-blind, placebo-controlled trial of donepezil hydrochloride (Aricept) for reducing the incidence of postoperative delirium after elective total hip replacement. *Int J Geriatr Psychiatry* 2007;22:343–349.

46. van Eijk MM, Roes KC, Honing ML, et al. Effect of rivastigmine as an adjunct to usual care with haloperidol on duration of delirium and mortality in critically ill patients: A multicentre, double-blind, placebo-controlled randomised trial. *Lancet* 2010;376:1829–1837.

47. Overshott R, Karim S, Burns A. Cholinesterase inhibitors for delirium. *Cochrane Database Syst Rev* 2008;(1):CD005317.

48. Chester JG, Rudolph JL. Vital signs in older patients: Age-related changes. *J Am Med Dir Assoc* 2011;12:337–343.

49. Chester JG, Harrington MB, Rudolph JL. Serial administration of a modified Richmond Agitation and Sedation Scale for delirium screening. *J Hosp Med* 2012;7(5):450–453.
50. *Diagnostic and Statistical Manual of Mental Disorders—III Revised*. Washington, DC: American Psychiatric Association, 1987.
51. Inouye SK, van Dyck CH, Alessi CA, Balkin S, Siegal AP, Horwitz RI. Clarifying confusion: The confusion assessment method. A new method for detection of delirium. *Ann Intern Med* 1990;113:941–948.
52. Wei LA, Fearing MA, Sternberg EJ, Inouye SK. The Confusion Assessment Method: A systematic review of current usage. *J Am Geriatr Soc* 2008;56:823–830.
53. O'Keeffe ST, Gosney MA. Assessing attentiveness in older hospital patients: Global assessment versus tests of attention. *J Am Geriatr Soc* 1997;45(4):470–473.
54. Stavros KA, Rudolph JL, Jones RN, Marcantonio ER. Delirium and the clinical assessment of attention in older adults. *J Am Geriatr Soc* 2008;56:S199–S200.
55. Ely EW, Margolin R, Francis J, May L, Truman B, Dittus R, et al. Evaluation of delirium in critically ill patients: Validation of the Confusion Assessment Method for the Intensive Care Unit (CAM-ICU). *Crit Care Med* 2001;29:1370–1379.
56. Pun BT, Ely EW. The importance of diagnosing and managing ICU delirium. *Chest* 2007;132:624–636.
57. Ely EW, Gautam S, Margolin R, Francis J, May L, Speroff T, et al. The impact of delirium in the intensive care unit on hospital length of stay. *Intensive Care Med* 2001;27: 1892–1900.
58. Milbrandt EB, Deppen S, Harrison PL, Shintani AK, Speroff T, Stiles RA, et al. Costs associated with delirium in mechanically ventilated patients. *Crit Care Med* 2004;32: 955–962.
59. Ely EW, Truman B, Shintani A, Thomason JW, Wheeler AP, Gordon S, et al. Monitoring sedation status over time in ICU patients: Reliability and validity of the Richmond Agitation-Sedation Scale (RASS). *JAMA* 2003;289:2983–2991.
60. Hart RP, Levenson JL, Sessler CN, Best AM, Schwartz SM, Rutherford LE. Validation of a cognitive test for delirium in medical ICU patients. *Psychosomatics* 1996;37: 533–546.
61. Alsop DC, Fearing MA, Johnson K, Sperling R, Fong TG, Inouye SK. The role of neuroimaging in elucidating delirium pathophysiology. *J Gerontol A Biol Sci Med Sci* 2006;61:1287–1293.
62. Breitbart W, Marotta R, Platt MM, Weisman H, Derevenco M, Grau C, et al. A double-blind trial of haloperidol, chlorpromazine, and lorazepam in the treatment of delirium in hospitalized AIDS patients. *Am J Psychiatry* 1996;153:231–237.
63. Campbell N, Boustani MA, Ayub A, Fox GC, Munger SL, Ott C, et al. Pharmacological management of delirium in hospitalized adults—A systematic evidence review. *J Gen Intern Med* 2009;24:848–853.
64. Schneider LS, Dagerman KS, Insel P. Risk of death with atypical antipsychotic drug treatment for dementia: Meta-analysis of randomized placebo-controlled trials. *JAMA* 2005;294:1934–1943.
65. Wang PS, Schneeweiss S, Avorn J, Fischer MA, Mogun H, Solomon DH, et al. Risk of death in elderly users of conventional vs. atypical antipsychotic medications. *N Engl J Med* 2005;353:2335–2341.
66. *Consensus Statement on High-Dose Antipsychotic Medication*. London, UK: Royal College of Psychiatrists, 2006.
67. Rudolph JL, Gardner KF, Gramigna GD, McGlinchey RE. Antipsychotics and oropharyngeal dysphagia in hospitalized older patients. *J Clin Psychopharmacol* 2008;28: 532–535.

68. Kiely DK, Marcantonio ER, Inouye SK, Shaffer ML, Bergmann MA, Yang FM, et al. Persistent delirium predicts greater mortality. *J Am Geriatr Soc* 2009;57:55–61.

69. Kiely DK, Jones RN, Bergmann MA, Murphy KM, Orav EJ, Marcantonio ER. Association between delirium resolution and functional recovery among newly admitted post-acute facility patients. *J Gerontol A Biol Sci Med Sci* 2006;61:204–208.

70. Fong TG, Jones RN, Shi P, Marcantonio ER, Yap L, Rudolph JL, et al. Delirium accelerates cognitive decline in Alzheimer disease. *Neurology* 2009;72:1570–1575.

71. Jones C, Griffiths RD, Humphris G, Skirrow PM. Memory, delusions, and the development of acute posttraumatic stress disorder-related symptoms after intensive care. *Crit Care Med* 2001;29:573–580.

72. Jones C, Backman C, Capuzzo M, Flaatten H, Rylander C, Griffiths RD. Precipitants of post-traumatic stress disorder following intensive care: A hypothesis generating study of diversity in care. *Intensive Care Med* 2007;33:978–985.

73. Rudolph JL, Inouye SK, Jones RN, Yang FM, Fong TG, Levkoff SE, et al. Delirium: An independent predictor of functional decline after cardiac surgery. *J Am Geriatr Soc* 2010;58:643–649.

74. Marcantonio ER, Flacker JM, Michaels M, Resnick NM. Delirium is independently associated with poor functional recovery after hip fracture. *J Am Geriatr Soc* 2000; 48:618–624.

75. Zigmond AS, Snaith RP. The hospital anxiety and depression scale. *Acta Psychiatr Scand* 1983;67:361–370.

76. Cully JA, Gfeller JD, Heise RA, Ross MJ, Teal CR, Kunik ME. Geriatric depression, medical diagnosis, and functional recovery during acute rehabilitation. *Arch Phys Med Rehabil* 2005;86:2256–2260.

CHAPTER 13

TRANSITIONAL CARE PLANNING: ASSURING A SAFE DISCHARGE

Satyen Nichani
Darius Joshi
Christopher S. Kim

INTRODUCTION

Transitional care at the time of hospital discharge can be a complex process, where patients may be at risk for errors and complications during the immediate post-discharge period. Definitions related to transitional care are shown in Box 13.1. Transitions of care occur across many settings (Fig. 13.1). The purpose of this chapter is to describe some key issues that affect the quality of hospital discharges, highlight some best practices around transitional care, and give recommendations on implementing these practices.

Over 12 million adults aged 65 years or older were hospitalized in 2007 according to the National Hospital Discharge Survey [1]. Although this segment accounted for just 13% of the total population of the United States, it comprised more than a third of total annual hospital discharges and almost half of total hospital days. This pattern of healthcare utilization is projected to increase steadily in future years as the national age-adjusted death rate and life expectancy reach record historical lows and highs, respectively [2].

Care transitions are frequently associated with adverse patient outcomes. In a 2007 Agency for Healthcare Research and Quality survey of hospitalized patients, 44% of respondents reported that hospital units did not coordinate well when transferring patients from one unit to another [3]. Forster and colleagues reported that one in five discharges was complicated by an adverse outcome, where a third of these could have been prevented and another third could have been ameliorated [4]. In 2005, the Medicare Payment Advisory Commission found that 17.6% of hospital discharges resulted in a readmission within 30 days, accounting for $15 billion in

Hospitalists' Guide to the Care of Older Patients, Edited by Brent C. Williams, Preeti N. Malani, and David H. Wesorick.

BOX 13.1

TERMS AND DEFINITIONS [37, 38]

Transition of care (or patient care transition) refers to the movement of a patient between different locations or different levels of care in the same location. *Transitional care* describes the coordinated efforts that preserve healthcare continuity and communication as patients transfer across healthcare domains.

Care coordination refers to the interaction among healthcare providers to ensure optimal care for a patient. This involves an accurate and efficient relay of information from one patient care team to the next as the patient transitions from one healthcare setting to another.

Discharge planning refers to the patient-centered systematic process that involves an assessment of the patient's needs and preparedness prior to hospital discharge, and the coordinated multidisciplinary activities that permit the delivery of appropriate postdischarge care in a safe environment.

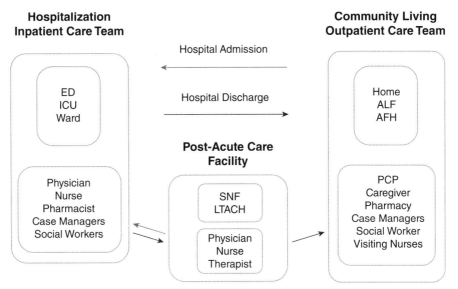

Figure 13.1   Care transitions between community-based and hospital-based care. A leftward arrow represents hospital admission and a rightward arrow represents patient discharge. ED, emergency department; ICU, intensive care unit; SNF, skilled nursing facility; LTACH, long-term acute care hospital; ALF, assisted living facility; AFH, adult foster home; PCP, primary care provider.

Medicare costs [5]. While not all readmissions are avoidable, these studies have resulted in increased attention to the discharge process.

WHY ARE HOSPITAL DISCHARGES CHALLENGING?

Many of the challenges in achieving quality care transitions from the hospital can be understood by examining the context in which these transitions occur.

The current reimbursement model does not provide incentives to healthcare organizations or individual providers to optimize the quality of hospital discharges. The Prospective Payment System and the adoption of a diagnosis-related group-based reimbursement for hospital-based care have resulted in increased efforts to reduce hospital lengths-of-stay [6]. This has led to older patients being more rapidly discharged from the hospital, potentially leading to more complex discharge plans.

The rapid growth of the hospitalist model of inpatient care in the United States has accentuated the discontinuity between inpatient and outpatient care, and increased the need for close communication between inpatient and outpatient providers. Unfortunately, while this need is well-recognized, direct communication between hospital physicians and primary care providers (PCPs) occurs infrequently, with an overreliance on indirect communication methods, such as written discharge summaries. A systematic review showed that only 3% of PCPs reported being involved in discussions about their patient's discharge, and only 20% reported being notified about the discharge [7]. The availability of a discharge summary at the patient's first postdischarge follow-up visit was also low (12–34%).

The hospital discharge is also complicated by a high frequency of medication-related errors and discrepancies. It is often difficult to ascertain the exact medications that a patient is taking at the time of hospital admission [8]. In one study of older patients admitted to a general medicine ward, at least one unintended medication discrepancy was found at the time of hospital admission in half of the cases, and a third of those were judged to have potential for causing patient discomfort or clinical deterioration [9]. The most common error was an omission of a medication taken regularly at home. Medication errors also occur because of inadequate care coordination during patient transitions within the hospital, such as when patients who were initially admitted to the intensive care unit are subsequently transferred to a lower level of care [10]. Contributing factors to such errors include a focus on acute care (with the temporary modification or discontinuation of many medications for chronic conditions), and lack of an organized hand-off process between care teams at the time of patient transfer. In addition, hospital formulary restrictions may require an automatic substitution of a medication with another of the same class during the patient's stay. These factors increase the risk of discrepancies in the patient's medication list at discharge, which occur in up to half of patients, and may result in adverse drug effects and avoidable healthcare utilization [11, 12].

The need to engage and partner with patients and their caregivers is also critical during the discharge transitions process. Patients (or their caregivers) may need to master a large amount of information in order adequately manage their own care after discharge, yet are often unable to list their medical diagnoses, or the names, purpose, or side effects of their medications [13]. This knowledge gap can result from both teaching problems and learning problems. Discharge teaching can be adversely affected by a lack of time or technical skills, and many patients have difficulty learning the discharge information. A large number of adults over 60 years have inadequate health literacy and read at approximately a third-grade level, yet reading materials given to patient are often written at or above an eleventh-grade level [14]. Many elders are also unable to read basic items, such as prescription bottles and appointment slips. Ethnic differences also exist, and a greater number of Spanish-speaking patients have inadequate health literacy compared with English speakers [15]. The high prevalence of low health literacy among elders, coupled with their chronic medical conditions and physical disabilities, makes it more difficult for them to participate in their own care.

BEST PRACTICES AROUND CARE TRANSITIONS AT HOSPITAL DISCHARGE

Optimal discharge planning requires robust incorporation of the following three processes: The *comprehensive assessment* of the patient's needs through a coordinated and multidisciplinary approach to engage the patient and caregiver in the transitions process; identification of the *best solutions* to meet postdischarge care needs; and the creation of a *systematic discharge process* that fosters the seamless transition of care.

Comprehensive Needs Assessment

It is important to perform a diligent assessment of the patient's postdischarge needs. Errors in the assessment of a patient's needs are certain to result in an inadequate discharge plan. Table 13.1 lists several questions that explore the patient's medical needs, functional status, psychological and cognitive state, caregiver support, and logistical and financial issues that influence the discharge process. There are several tools that can assist with this

TABLE 13.1 Questions Involved in the Comprehensive Assessment of a Patient's Discharge Needs [36]

Assess the patient's medical needs
• Will the patient have new medications, treatments, or devices after discharge (e.g., parenteral medications, wound care, etc.)?

Assess the patient's mobility and functional status
• Can the patient perform ADLs, IADLs, and medical treatments (as above)? Will the patient need assistance after discharge?
• Has the patient been assessed by Physical and/or Occupational Therapy?
• Does the patient have limiting sensory deficits (e.g., deafness or blindness)?

Assess the patient's psychological/cognitive state
• Does the patient have cognitive impairment or difficulty with medical decision making?
• What is the patient's level of health literacy?
• Does the patient have a mood disorder or difficulty with behavioral control that is impacting his health?
• Does the patient have issues with substance abuse or dependence?

Assess the patient's caregiver support
• If the patient cannot care for himself, who will provide care? Are the identified caregivers able to care for the patient, given the needs identified above?

Assess for logistical or financial issues
• Is the patient's prehospital living situation adequate or will he need an alternative living situation at the time of discharge?
• Is the patient's prior mode of community dwelling inaccessible? For example, is the patient able to climb the flight of stairs needed to enter his apartment?
• Does the patient have adequate transportation to follow-up appointments and services?
• Is the patient experiencing financial difficulty and/or inadequate insurance coverage for medications and services?

ADL, activity of daily living; IADL, instrumental activity of daily living.

assessment. A few examples of recommended tools are listed in Table 13.2, and several of these are discussed in greater detail in Chapter 3.

Assessment of a patient's discharge needs often requires a multidisciplinary team of health professionals, each of whom may have relevant but separate pieces of information about a patient's condition. Some of the common functions of the members of the discharge planning team are shown in Table 13.3. Because of differences in available resources, job descriptions, and local culture, the composition of the discharge team may vary significantly between hospitals. In fact, it is also common for the team members to have overlapping roles. Ideally, patients and families should also be considered key members of this team.

TABLE 13.2   Examples of Assessment Tools to Evaluate a Patient's Discharge Needs

Parameter	Example	Description/Comments
Functional status	Katz ADL Scale	Evaluates the activities of daily living by assessing the patient's level of independence or dependence in the following activities: bathing, dressing, toileting, transferring, continence, and feeding.
	Lawton IADL Scale	Evaluates the instrumental activities of daily living by assessing the patient's ability to function in the following domains: ability to use the telephone, shopping, food preparation, housekeeping, laundry, transportation, responsibility for own medications, and ability to handle finances.
Mobility	Timed Up and Go (TUG) test	Evaluates the patient's ability to stand up from sitting in a chair, walk 3 m, turn, and return to the chair.
Hearing impairment	Whisper voice test	Assesses the patient's hearing by speaking and whispering a set of three random numbers at 6 in and 2 ft from the ear.
Psychological state	Mini-Mental State Examination (MMSE)	Widely used measure of cognitive impairment but scores may be influenced by education level and cultural back ground
	Mini-COG test	Measure of cognitive impairment; uses a three-item recall test and a scored clock-drawing test. Scores relatively unaffected by ethnicity, language and education
	Five-item Geriatric Depression Scale (GDS)	Measures responses to five questions that screen for depression
Health Literacy	Rapid Estimate of Adult Literacy in Medicine, Revised (REALM-R)	Word recognition test consisting of 11 items used to identify people at risk for poor health literacy.

TABLE 13.3   Members of a Multidisciplinary Discharge Team and a Brief Description of Their Roles

Member	Roles (may overlap)
Physician	• Assess and discuss with patient/caregiver details of patient's medical condition (including prognosis). • Seek patient preferences and choices • Determine goals of care for current hospitalization and need for postdischarge care/services. • Determine readiness for discharge and notify patient/ caregivers of discharge date. • Educate patient/caregiver and discuss postdischarge plan of care in a manner that is commensurate with the individual's level of health literacy. • Communicate and coordinate follow-up care with outpatient providers. • Arrange for necessary postdischarge care/services. • Remain available to assist and troubleshoot post-discharge problems.
Nurse	• Patient teaching (e.g., wound care instructions, skill for self-injection of medications). • Provide patient/caregiver with discharge instruction sheet and confirm understanding by the teach-back process. • Confirm transportation arrangements.
Discharge planner	• Contact patient/caregiver to confirm discharge date and transportation arrangements. • Establish that the patient's discharge destination is safe and accessible. • Confirm arrangements for durable medical equipment and home supplies and confirm availability of necessary home services. • When transferring/discharging to another facility, seek patient/family preference and make necessary referrals.
Social worker	• Identify patient's financial status and coverage for services, including medications. • Assist patients with social and emotional needs such as coping with traumatic or chronic illnesses, alcoholism, and substance abuse, marital difficulties due to illness, adult abuse and domestic violence, bereavement and work-related concerns. • Assist patients and families with advance directives, living will, durable power of attorney, guardianship, and identification of patient's next of kin. • Provide patients with details of available community resources.

(Continued)

TABLE 13.3 (*Continued*)

Member	Roles (may overlap)
Physical and occupational therapist	• Evaluate patient's level of functional independence including mobility. • Make appropriate recommendations for equipment needs, such as ambulation devices, and that needed for self-care and independence with ADLs. • Instruct patient/caregiver in proper transfers and positioning techniques and facilitate optimal safety and independence. Instruct patients/caregiver in use and appropriate maintenance of orthotic devices. • Make recommendations for follow-up physical and occupational therapy, and location of services such as subacute rehabilitation facility, home therapy, or outpatient therapy.
Nutritionist	• Assess patient's nutritional needs and make dietary recommendations to the patient/caregiver. • Make recommendations for enteral and parenteral nutritional therapy in patients unable to tolerate or maintain adequate oral intake. • Educate and provide nutritional information for special patient populations, for example, patients on renal replacement therapy, diabetics, vitamin K antagonist (warfarin), and electrolyte disturbances.
Pharmacist	• Assist medical staff with drug regimens, drug profile and interactions (drug–drug, drug–patient). • Assist with medication reconciliation at hospital admission and discharge. • Provide patient/caregiver with information on new and important medications.
Discharge advocate and complex case manager	• Collaborate with healthcare providers to advocate for the well-being of patients with complex medical illness and needs.

A discharge team that meets regularly for discharge rounds offers several advantages. Gathered professionals are able to share their perspectives, build consensus regarding patient management, divide responsibilities based on individual expertise, and remain consistent in their communications with patients and caregivers. At the core of the discharge planning team is the role of the case manager. Case managers collaborate closely with the other members of the discharge planning team and serve as liaisons between patients and their families and outside agencies, such as nursing homes, medical equipment providers, and payers.

Some patients may be at particularly high risk for adverse events related to the hospital discharge. Several risk assessment tools have been studied as potential predictors of unplanned hospital readmissions [16]. Unfortunately, risk assessment tools have demonstrated limited ability to predict which patients are at high risk for readmission. Perhaps a better way to evaluate the available risk assessment tools may be to utilize them to identify which patients may require additional services and enhanced care coordination by the multidisciplinary discharge team. A readily available tool is the Society of Hospital Medicine's Project BOOST (Better Outcomes for Older Adults through Safe Transitions) 8P scoring system (problem medications, psychological barriers, principal diagnosis, polypharmacy, poor health literacy, patient support, prior hospitalization, and palliative care), which can be applied to patients throughout their hospital stay to identify potential barriers to a safe discharge [17].

Identifying Solutions and the Appropriate Level of Postdischarge Care

For successful discharge planning, it is important to develop solutions that match the patient's needs with appropriate resources and preserve the patient's autonomy and the family's well-being. Finding the right solutions requires an experienced team that possesses a solid understanding of the available local resources.

A crucial aspect in the proper delivery of postdischarge services is identifying the appropriate location (site) of such care. This decision must take into consideration the intensity of treatment that will be necessary after discharge, the level of support that the patient will require, the patient's prognosis for improvement, and the patient's long-term care needs. Figure 13.2 shows a schematic of the types of postdischarge care that are available.

Understanding Posthospital Care Options   Posthospital care can be broadly divided into "skilled" and "unskilled" services. Skilled services may include varying degrees of nursing care, physical therapy (PT), occupational therapy (OT), and speech therapy. Some patients stand to benefit from facility-based care (e.g., acute rehabilitation, or subacute care in a skilled nursing facility), while others might be best cared for at home by visiting nurses and therapists. For the elderly, posthospitalization skilled care is a Medicare Part A benefit (akin to hospital care). Other older adults may stand to benefit from "unskilled" services in long-term care facilities that can provide additional supervision and assistance. These long-term options

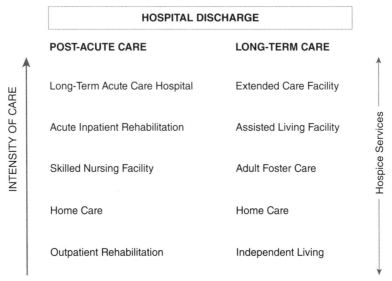

Figure 13.2   Posthospital care options arranged by service intensity.

provide varying degrees of day-to-day support and assistance. A brief summary of various posthospital care options is provided here.

Post-Acute (Skilled) Care Options

Long-Term Acute Care Hospital (LTACH)   These units provide highly specialized care to patients with complex medical and surgical conditions that require extended hospital-level inpatient care. The Centers for Medicare and Medicaid Services defines a LTACH as a hospital that has an average length of stay of greater than 25 days. These units utilize a multi-disciplinary team of physicians, nurses, respiratory therapists, pharmacists, and rehabilitation therapists. Examples of patients who require such care include those with tracheostomies requiring a high-level of pulmonary toileting, those requiring a slow wean or extended mechanical ventilation, a high level of supplemental oxygen (greater than 5 L/min), or those needing cardiac telemetric monitoring. Following stabilization, patients from LTACHs often transition to subacute care for continued rehabilitation and nursing care.

Acute (Inpatient) Rehabilitation Hospitals   These skilled care areas are designed for patients who would benefit from intensive, short-term rehabilitation under the direct supervision of Physical Medicine and Rehabilitation physicians (physiatrists). To qualify for payments under Medicare, patients must be able to participate in at least 3 hours per day of PT and OT and demonstrate progress. Unfortunately, elders are often unable to tolerate this intensity of therapy after hospital discharge due to their compromised physical endurance and complex medical issues.

Subacute Care   Subacute care represents a niche of post-acute care along the continuum between acute-hospital care and long-term nursing home care [18]. Examples of subacute care services include continued treatment of partially resolved acute conditions, management of coexisting problems and comorbidities, delivery of rehabilitative care, and skilled nursing care, such as parenteral antibiotics or wound care, that no longer requires hospitalization. Subacute care is a Medicare Part A and private insurance benefit that allows for medical, nursing, and rehabilitative care of patients who cannot safely be cared for in the home environment.

The vast majority of subacute care is done in Skilled Nursing Facilities (SNFs). These facilities have to be certified by Medicare to provide posthospital care under Medicare. Medicare Part A typically allows for a maximum of 100 days of care in a SNF if the patient meets skilled nursing and rehabilitation criteria. If the 100 days of SNF benefits is "exhausted," it may be renewed if the Medicare recipient is able to stay outside of all Medicare facilities for a full 60 days after discharge. For a patient with Medicare as the sole insurer, a patient copayment begins after day 20 in the SNF. The copayment percentage further increases on days 40 and 60. If available, secondary insurers often cover such Medicare mandated copayments. For a patient to be admitted for subacute care at an SNF, Medicare requires a minimum of three nights of hospital stay within the previous 30 days. Patients in a SNF typically (but not always) are able to tolerate between 1 and 3 hours of PT, OT, and speech therapies for 5 days per week. The average length of stay for subacute care in a SNF is between 20 and 25 days [19].

Skilled Homecare   Skilled homecare (often termed Home Health Care) is a Medicare Part A and private insurance benefit for patients who are discharged from the hospital, acute rehabilitation unit, LTACH, or subacute care who need ongoing nursing care, OT, or PT in their home environment. Medicare requires that patients be mostly homebound (except for physician visits) to qualify for these services. The level, frequency, and intensity of skilled homecare are determined by the patient's skilled nursing and therapy needs and monitored by Medicare and private payers. Skilled homecare is one of the fastest growing Medicare Part A benefits.

Long-Term Care Options
Nursing Home/Extended Care Facility (ECF)   The majority of the patients who live in a nursing home have severe cognitive, neurological,

or other physical disabilities leading to long-term functional impairment necessitating continuous nursing care. For the majority of these patients, the nursing home is their "home" for the remaining duration of their lives. This type of "long-term" nursing home care should not be confused with short-term subacute care, which may be provided to patients within the same nursing home and sometimes on the same unit within the nursing home. Long-term nursing home care is paid for by private funds, long-term care insurance, Medicaid (for qualified indigent residents in some states), or the Veterans Administration. Medicare (Part A or B) does not pay for any of these long term care options. Some nursing homes offer specialized and secure units for persons with dementia. These specialized "dementia units" allow for greater independence in ambulation (wandering), dignified care, and increased supervision for this population.

Assisted Living Facilities (ALF)   Assisted Living Facilities provide a home-like living environment that offer varying degrees of additional support. They serve a less disabled clientele than ECFs, and some also offer specialized units for persons with dementia. Support in the form of health aides and nursing care is available. Examples of such assistance include medication dispensing and closer supervision for the cognitively impaired. Patients are housed in self-contained units that include living quarters and a private bathroom. As the cost of ECFs has increased, ALFs are caring for a greater number of persons with higher levels of cognitive and physical disabilities. Some state Medicaid programs provide for a limited amount of assisted living coverage for the indigent elderly.

Adult Foster Care (AFC)   Residents in this small group living setting are cared for by nonclinically trained, private caregivers in private homes. Most residents are elderly or disabled. Additional nursing services are not available on site but can be hired. Many offer medication dispensing and assistance with ADLs. Residents may have their own rooms or share them. The elderly and their families often choose this option of care when they cannot afford the higher monthly expense of an ALF or ECF.

Other Options
Hospice Services   Hospice provides supportive and palliative care for patients who are near the end of their lives (e.g., those patients with an estimated life expectancy of less than 6 months). These services can be provided in any long term care setting, but are most often provided in the patient's home (supported by family members or caregivers) or in a hospice facility (residential hospice). Treatments that are considered curative are usually not

covered by insurance for hospice patients. Hospice care is covered by Medicare but patients are required to pay for room and board, as applicable.

Continuing Care Retirement Community (CCRC)   Also referred to as "life care communities," these campuses include independent living apartments, assisted living, and nursing homes that provide a continuum of residential and service options that are able to meet an individual's needs in keeping with the principle of "aging in place." Such a model of care may appeal to those living independently who are reluctant to move. Residents of CCRCs are able to easily transition back and forth between different levels of care. For example, a resident in independent living may transition to an assisted living unit or a skilled nursing facility for a few days until they have gained complete recovery from an acute illness prior to returning to their previous independent arrangement. This model also suits couples who differ in their health needs and reside in different facilities within the same campus while remaining close to each other.

Building a Systematic Discharge Process

Even though every patient is unique, several common elements are incorporated into every hospital discharge. We believe that hospitalists can improve their discharge process by adhering to the following five principles:

1. *Reconcile medications carefully.* Diligent medication reconciliation at the time of discharge should be carefully performed, comparing the discharge medication list to both inpatient and home medication lists. Special attention should be paid to potential drug–drug interactions and drug classes associated with a higher likelihood of adverse drug effects, such as antiplatelet agents, anticoagulants, insulin and oral hypoglycemic agents, antiarrhythmic, and immunosuppressive drugs. Hospital pharmacists are not only able to help with medication assessment and reconciliation, but can also assist with medication adherence screening and patient education, thereby reducing medication discrepancies [20, 21]. Hospitals should also work toward adopting an institution-wide systematic method that permits comparison of all inpatient medications to the patient's home list at any time during the hospital stay. More information about medication reconciliation in older patients can be found in Chapter 6.

2. *Collaborate closely with primary care physicians.* When possible, hospitalists should collaborate with PCPs in developing an appropriate treatment and discharge plan. Not only are PCPs familiar with

the patient's past history, but they may also be aware of previous treatment preferences made by the patient. Direct communication also serves to provide the PCP with important information (that can supplement a written summary), and allows the PCP to ask specific questions.

3. *Arrange for postdischarge follow-up.* Collaboration with PCPs also carries the added benefit of timely postdischarge follow-up. Primary care continuity after discharge has been associated with a reduced risk of urgent readmission and death at 6 months [22]. Appointment times should be made in consultation with the patient and caregivers to maximize compliance.

4. *Produce a high-quality discharge summary.* The discharge summary is an indirect but common method used by hospital-based providers to communicate with PCPs and other healthcare providers outside of the hospital system. The quality, accuracy, and timeliness of the discharge summary are important considerations. Table 13.4 lists some of the characteristics of a high-quality discharge summary.

TABLE 13.4   Characteristics of a High-Quality Discharge Summary [23, 39]

- Structured format
- Concise (less than two pages length except as needed for complex patients)
- Timely
- Accurate
- Preferred content:
    1. Discharge diagnoses (primary and secondary)
    2. Discharge medications (complete list rather than a limited list of only medication changes)
    3. Brief description of the hospital course
    4. Recommendations of any subspecialty consultants
    5. List of active medical conditions at discharge
    6. Arranged medical follow-up appointments (including time and location)
    7. Aspects of medical care or social issues pending at the time of discharge
    8. Important information about pending laboratory tests and investigations
    9. Patient prognosis
    10. Discharge location
    11. Overview of postdischarge community services
    12. Identification of referring and receiving providers
    13. Any anticipated problems and suggested interventions
    14. A 24/7 call-back number.

Van Walraven and colleagues found that PCPs preferred the inclusion of both normal and abnormal clinical findings and laboratory values pertinent to the patient's condition as compared with the inclusion of only abnormal findings [23]. PCPs also preferred a summary of the results of major investigations (as opposed to complete reports), and that discharge summaries be kept concise and follow a structured format (as opposed to a narrative or letter style). The reproduction of a detailed description of the patient's prehospital course in the discharge summary is not required when the patient's diagnosis is clear.

5. *Provide clear discharge instructions appropriate to the patient's level of health literacy, and assess the patient's understanding of these instructions.* Key aspects involved in effectively communicating with patients include language (avoiding jargon and speaking in terms that the patient understands), pragmatism (providing a plan that the patient can follow), and patience (spending a reasonable amount of time counseling the patient and verifying their comprehension of discharge instructions). Patients and caregivers should be educated about condition-specific issues, such as pain management, wound care, dietary modifications, and any necessary limitations in activity or duties at work. They should be alerted to red flags or warning symptoms that should prompt appropriate medical attention, as well as instructions on how to act and whom to contact. A contact number and names of available providers should be included in their discharge instructions.

Teaching sessions should be scheduled at times that are convenient for the patient, when they are alert and interested in participating, in the company of their caregivers. The teach-back method, in which physicians ask the patient to restate instructions or information to ensure that they were correctly understood and remembered, is an important strategy in improving physician-patient communication, and its use has been associated with improved outcomes [24]. The teach-back has subsequently evolved to also include "show-back" (i.e., the patient demonstrates the procedures that he or she will need to carry out after discharge). And while the patient's ability to "teach-back" or "show-back" does not guarantee full comprehension, it provides a practical approach to dynamically engage with the patient about their own care, which can be reinforced in future visits. Lastly, hospital-based practitioners should provide clear answers to questions, provide comfort and reassurance, and include these instructions in the discharge summary (or a written patient-centered discharge document), a copy of which should always be given to patients at the time of discharge. Important elements should be highlighted, and the print should be large enough to be read by patients (a font size of at least 14 points is desirable).

Combining easy-to-read written materials with oral instructions also greatly enhances patient understanding. The use of nonwritten materials such as picture books also benefits patients by increasing attention, comprehension, and recall of health information, especially in those with low literacy skills [25]. The use of videotapes, television, and other media-based educational tools has also been shown to improve patients' short-term knowledge [26].

A separate patient-centered discharge document is a valuable complement to the verbal instructions given to patients at the time of discharge. Unlike the discharge summary that is often generated for use by health professionals, this document's structure and style should be developed for use by patients and does not require a presumed level of medical understanding. Such a document utilizes elements that appeal to the patient's interest, such as well-defined sections with bold-faced headers and suitable fonts and color coding. These documents can also incorporate visual elements, such as tables, figures, and calendars where necessary. Simplicity is a critical feature and care should be taken to minimize information overload. Other elements central to this document include the following:

- A simplistic description of the discharge diagnoses enhanced by the use of illustrations and associated printouts of pertinent, patient-centered, condition-specific health information.
- Names and contact information of all relevant healthcare professionals.
- Dates, locations, and reasons for postdischarge appointments and tests.
- A medication schedule that also includes a separate listing of new and discontinued medications and medication dose changes, primary indication for each medication, and a list of important adverse effects for the patient to monitor.
- Information about recommended steps the patient should take if a problem arises.

The "after-hospital care plan" by Project RED (Re-Engineered Discharge) is an example of such a document that can be accessed at http://www.bu.edu/fammed/projectred/toolkit.html. The use of a patient-centered discharge document has been associated with a higher rate of patient reported self-preparedness, knowledge of discharge diagnosis, and postdischarge follow-up visits [27].

POSTDISCHARGE INTERVENTIONS

Several innovative postdischarge interventions have been studied. Many of these interventions have resulted in some success, although it is not always clear which element of the intervention provided benefit, or if the intervention is cost-effective.

Some studies have attempted to improve the discharge process through the use of discharge advocates (or *transition coaches*). These trained professionals, often nurses who are familiar with the patient's condition and care during their hospital stay, function to coordinate care across the care continuum and provide support to older patients and their caregivers in the immediate postdischarge period [27–30]. Their work combines tasks that are traditionally performed by several professionals into a single role. They assist with several critical aspects of the discharge process including educating patients and caregivers, medication reconciliation, developing patient-centered discharge documents, communicating and transmitting discharge summaries to primary care providers, arranging follow-up appointments and visits, making postdischarge follow-up home visits or telephone calls, communicating test results, and ensuring treatment adherence.

Complex case managers are another type of professional involved in bridging care across multiple hospital admissions and discharges. They work with high-risk patients (especially those with frequent hospital readmissions and those with persistent barriers, such as substance abuse, behavioral problems, or medical noncompliance) on an outpatient basis for extended periods.

Postdischarge telephone calls are another way to try to bridge patients across the discharge transition. These calls serve to assess the patient's progress, reinforce the doctor–patient relationship, provide an opportunity to answer questions, and bolster treatment adherence. Besides physicians, some practices have used nurses, pharmacists, and other medical providers to make these calls. Familiarity with the patient and personal knowledge of their problems during their hospitalization, a previous rapport, and the timing of the follow-up telephone call (within 1 week of discharge, ideally within 72 hours) are factors that directly impact the value of these calls [31].

A *hospitalist-led post-discharge clinic* is another possible intervention to bolster the quality of transitional care after discharge. Besides addressing several issues similar to postdischarge telephone contact, these "bridge" clinics allow for timely reevaluation of patients after hospital discharge. However, these clinics are often difficult to fund and staff. Other barriers include the possibility of "responsibility creep" that requires hospitalists to extend their responsibility out of the hospital, and high patient "no-show" rates [32, 33]. These clinics are especially valuable for bridging the care of those patients who either cannot get in to see their PCPs or have no established PCP.

While anecdotal evidence suggests that patients find these postdischarge interventions extremely valuable, the impact of these interventions on readmission rates, postdischarge healthcare utilization, medication discrepancies, and cost have varied in prospective studies [20, 27–29, 34]. With policy efforts to support a bundled payment system that pays for "episodes of care" including postdischarge acute care services, hospitals may show an even greater interest in developing similar effective postdischarge interventions in the future [35].

CONCLUSION

The hospital discharge is a transition of care that is both important and complicated. Table 13.5 summarizes the salient features of a robust discharge process. While it is agreed that all the elements of the discharge process are valuable, it is very important to realize that there does not appear to be a "one-size fits all" recipe for effective discharge planning. Hospitalists should strive to perform a thorough review of the patient's needs and choose solutions that best match the patient's needs and preferences.

TABLE 13.5 Summary of Recommended Interventions that Hospitalists Should Consistently Adopt to Improve the Quality of Hospital Discharges

1. Perform a systematic, comprehensive needs assessment that explores the patient's medical, functional, psychological/cognitive, and social domains with input from a multidisciplinary discharge team that meets regularly for discharge planning rounds.
2. Seek the patient's perspective and treatment preferences and develop a mutually acceptable discharge plan.
3. Perform a risk assessment for postdischarge complications on a per-patient basis.
4. Assess the patient's health literacy that should guide communication and patient education.
5. Perform a diligent reconciliation of the patient's medications and prospectively explore barriers to discharge medication coverage and accessibility.
6. Educate patients and caregivers in a manner that incorporates patient engagement and assess the degree of understanding by the teach-back process.
7. Effectively communicate and coordinate care with primary care providers and arrange for timely postdischarge follow-up.
8. Produce high-quality discharge summaries and patient-centered discharge documents.
9. Bolster the discharge process, especially for high-risk patients, via postdischarge telephone calls, utilizing discharge advocates, or involving complex care managers.

ADDITIONAL RESOURCES

National collaborative efforts such as the Society of Hospital Medicine's mentored implementation program called Project BOOST (http://www.hospitalmedicine.org/boost/) [36], and multidisciplinary groups such as the National Transitions of Care Coalition (http://www.ntocc.org) offer a wide-array of resources that hospitalists may utilize to improve the quality of care transitions at their own hospital.

REFERENCES

1. Hall MJ, DeFrances CJ, Williams SN, Golosinskiy A, Schwartzman A. National hospital discharge survey: 2007 summary. *Natl Health Stat Report* 2010;29:1–20, 24.
2. Xu J, Kochanek KD, Murphy SL, Tejada-Vera B *Deaths: Final Data for 2007*. National vital statistics reports. Hyattsville, MD: National Center for Health Statistics, 2010.
3. Agency for Healthcare Quality and Research. Hospital survey on patient safety culture: 2007 comparative database report. AHRQ Publication No. 07-0025. 2007: Available at: http://www.ahrq.gov/qual/hospsurveydb/ (accessed April 11, 2013).
4. Forster AJ, Murff HJ, Peterson JF, Gandhi TK, Bates DW. The incidence and severity of adverse events affecting patients after discharge from the hospital. *Ann Intern Med* 2003;138:161–174.
5. The Medicare Payment Advisory Commission. Report to the congress: Promoting greater efficiency in Medicare. Washington, DC. 2007. Available at: http://www.medpac.gov/documents/Jun07_EntireReport.pdf (accessed April 11, 2013).
6. Kosecoff J, Kahn KL, Rogers WH, Reinisch EJ, Sherwood MJ, Rubenstein LV, et al. Prospective payment system and impairment at discharge. The "quicker-and-sicker" story revisited. *JAMA* 1990;264(15):1980–1983.
7. Kripalani S, LeFevre F, Phillips CO, Williams MV, Basaviah P, Baker DW. Deficits in communication and information transfer between hospital-based and primary care physicians: Implications for patient safety and continuity of care. *JAMA* 2007;297(8):831–841.
8. Kessels RPC. Patients' memory for medical information. *J R Soc Med* 2003;96(5):219–222.
9. Cornish PL, Knowles SR, Marchesano R, Tam V, Shadowitz S, Juurlink DN, et al. Unintended medication discrepancies at the time of hospital admission. *Arch Intern Med* 2005;165(4):424–429.
10. Bell CM, Brener SS, Gunraj N, Huo C, Bierman AS, Scales DC, et al. Association of icu or hospital admission with unintentional discontinuation of medications for chronic diseases. *JAMA* 2011;306(8):840–847.
11. Moore C, Wisnivesky J, Williams S, McGinn T. Medical errors related to discontinuity of care from an inpatient to an outpatient setting. *J Gen Intern Med* 2003;18(8):646–651.
12. Schnipper JL, Kirwin JL, Cotugno MC, Wahlstrom SA, Brown BA, Tarvin E, et al. Role of pharmacist counseling in preventing adverse drug events after hospitalization. *Arch Intern Med* 2006;166(5):565–571.
13. Makaryus AN, Friedman Ea. Patients' understanding of their treatment plans and diagnosis at discharge. *Mayo Clin Proc* 2005;80(8):991–994.

14. Murphy PW, Davis TC, Jackson RH, Decker BC, Long SW. Effects of literacy on health care of the aged: Implications for health professionals. *Educ Gerontol* 1993;19(4): 311–316.

15. Gazmararian JA, Baker DW, Williams MV, Parker RM, Scott TL, Green DC, et al. Health literacy among Medicare enrollees in a managed care organization. *JAMA* 1999;281(6): 545–551.

16. Allaudeen N, Schnipper JL, Orav EJ, Wachter RM, Vidyarthi AR. Inability of providers to predict unplanned readmissions. *J Gen Intern Med* 2011.

17. Project BOOST. Risk assessment tool: The 8ps. Philadelphia: Society of Hospital Medicine; 2011. Available at: http://www.hospitalmedicine.org/ResourceRoomRedesign/RR_CareTransitions/html_CC/06Boost/03_Assessment.cfm (accessed April 11, 2013).

18. Lewin-VHI, Inc. *Subacute Care: Review of the Literature*. Washington, DC: U.S. Department of Health and Human Services, 1994.

19. von Sternberg T, Hepburn K, Cibuzar P, Convery L, Dokken B, Haefemeyer J, et al. Post-hospital sub-acute care: An example of a managed care model. *J Am Geriatr Soc* 1997 Jan;45(1):87–91.

20. Walker PC, Bernstein SJ, Jones JNT, Piersma J, Kim H-W, Regal RE, et al. Impact of a pharmacist-facilitated hospital discharge program: A quasi-experimental study. *Arch Intern Med* 2009;169(21):2003–2010.

21. Kaboli PJ, Hoth AB, McClimon BJ, Schnipper JL. Clinical pharmacists and inpatient medical care: A systematic review. *Arch Intern Med* 2006;166(9):955–964.

22. van Walraven C, Taljaard M, Etchells E, Bell CM, Stiell IG, Zarnke K, et al. The independent association of provider and information continuity on outcomes after hospital discharge: Implications for hospitalists. *J Hosp Med* 2010;5(7):398–405.

23. van Walraven C, Rokosh E. What is necessary for high-quality discharge summaries? *Am J Med Qual* 1999;14(4):160–169.

24. Schillinger D, Piette J, Grumbach K, Wang F, Wilson C, Daher C, et al. Closing the loop: Physician communication with diabetic patients who have low health literacy. *Arch Intern Med* 2003;163(1):83–90.

25. Houts PS, Doak CC, Doak LG, Loscalzo MJ. The role of pictures in improving health communication: A review of research on attention, comprehension, recall, and adherence. *Patient Educ Couns* 2006;61(2):173–190.

26. Health NWGoLa. Communicating with patients who have limited literacy skills. *J Fam Pract* 1998;46(2):168–176.

27. Jack BW, Chetty VK, Anthony D, Greenwald JL, Sanchez GM, Johnson AE, et al. A reengineered hospital discharge program to decrease rehospitalization: A randomized trial. *Ann Intern Med* 2009;150(3):178–187.

28. Naylor MD. Comprehensive discharge planning and home follow-up of hospitalized elders: A randomized clinical trial. *JAMA* 1999;281(7):613–620.

29. Coleman EA, Parry C, Chalmers S, Min S-J. The care transitions intervention: Results of a randomized controlled trial. *Arch Intern Med* 2006;166(17):1822–1828.

30. Finn KM, Heffner R, Chang Y, Bazari H, Hunt D, Pickell K, et al. Improving the discharge process by embedding a discharge facilitator in a resident team. *J Hosp Med* 2011;6(9): 494–500.

31. Bowman GS, Howden J, Allen S, Webster RA, Thompson DR. A telephone survey of medical patients 1 week after discharge from hospital. *J Clin Nurs* 1994;3(6): 369–373.

32. Beresford L. Is a post-discharge clinic in your hospital's future? *Hospitalist* 2011; 15:1, 34–36, 41–42.

33. Diem SJ, Prochazka AV, Meyer TJ, Fryer GE. Effects of a postdischarge clinic on houseestaff satisfaction and utilization of hospital services. *J Gen Intern Med* 1996;11(3): 179–181.

34. Nelson JR. The importance of postdischarge telephone follow-up for hospitalists: A view from the trenches. *Dis Mon* 2002;48(4):273–275.

35. Center for Medicare and Medicaid Innovation. *Bundled Payments for Care Improvement.* Baltimore, MD: Centers for Medicare & Medicaid Services, 2011. Available at: http://innovations.cms.gov/initiatives/bundled-payments/ (accessed April 11, 2013).

36. Society of Hospital Medicine. Boosting care transitions. Philadelphia: Society of Hospital Medicine; 2011. Available at: http://www.hospitalmedicine.org/ResourceRoomRedesign/RR_CareTransitions/html_CC/project_boost_background.cfm (accessed April 11, 2013).

37. Coleman EA, Berenson RA. Lost in transition: Challenges and opportunities for improving the quality of transitional care. *Ann Intern Med* 2004;141(7):533–536.

38. National Transitions of Care Coalition. Improving transitions of care. National Transitions of Care Coalition; 2010. Available at: http://www.ntocc.org/Portals/0/PDF/Resources/NTOCCIssueBriefs.pdf (accessed April 11, 2013).

39. Halasyamani L, Kripalani S, Coleman E, Schnipper J, van Walraven C, Nagamine J, et al. Transition of care for hospitalized elderly patients—development of a discharge checklist for hospitalists. *J Hosp Med* 2006;1(6):354–360.

INDEX

Note: Page numbers in *italics* indicate illustrations; tables are noted with *t*.

Abilify, for psychosis, 107*t*
Absorption of medications, 67–68
ACCP. *See* American College of Chest Physicians
ACE units. *See* Acute care of the elderly (ACE) units
Acetabulum, replacement of, 145
Acetaminophen, 207
Acetylcholine receptor, blockade of, mental status changes and, 95
Acetylcholinesterase inhibitors, delirium and, 211–212
ACOVE. *See* Assessing Care of Vulnerable Elders
Acromegaly, findings of classic facies, 9*t*
Activities of daily living, 1, 19, 21*t*, 26*t*
    baseline function and, 206
    nutrition and, 118
    questions about, at admission and during hospital stay, 22
Acute care hospitals
    pressure ulcers and, 181
    preventing, 182
Acute care model, 18
Acute care of the elderly (ACE) units, 20
Acute-on-chronic framework, for hospitalization among older patients, *19*
Acute rehabilitation hospitals, 234–235
Addison's disease, 8
ADEs. *See* Adverse drug events
ADLs. *See* Activities of daily living

Admission to hospital
    falls occurring during, 166–167
    medication errors and, 75
    reconciling medications at, 86
ADRs. *See* Adverse drug reactions
Adult foster care, 236
Adult foster home, *226*
Advance directives, 59–60
Adventitious movements, noting, 10
Adverse drug events, 1, 65
    in hospitals, 74–75
    reducing risk of, 83
    transitional care and, 75
Adverse drug reactions, 65
    in hospitals, 75
    prescribing cascades and, 71
AFH. *See* Adult foster home
African-Americans, end-of-life decision-making and, 42
After-hospital care plan, 240
Age, chronological *vs.* apparent, 8
Ageism, underrepresentation in clinical trials and, 66
Agency for Healthcare Research and Quality, survey of hospitalized patients, 225
Aging
    anthropometric measurements and, 116
    psychotropic medications and, 97
"Aging in place," 237
Agitation
    acute, treatments for, 110*t*–111*t*
    delirium-associated, management of, 217–218
    treating, 109

Hospitalists' Guide to the Care of Older Patients, Edited by Brent C. Williams, Preeti N. Malani, and David H. Wesorick.
© 2013 by John Wiley & Sons, Inc. Published 2013 by John Wiley & Sons, Inc.